SOAP MAKING RECIPES

Techniques and Recipes for Creating All Manner of Liquid and Soft Soap Naturally

(Organic Soap Making Procedure and Ingredients)

Julie Ford

Published by Oliver Leish

Julie Ford

All Rights Reserved

Soap Making Recipes: Techniques and Recipes for Creating All Manner of Liquid and Soft Soap Naturally (Organic Soap Making Procedure and Ingredients)

ISBN 978-1-77485-082-4

All rights reserved. No part of this guide may be reproduced in any form without permission in writing from the publisher except in the case of brief quotations embodied in critical articles or reviews.

Legal & Disclaimer

The information contained in this book is not designed to replace or take the place of any form of medicine or professional medical advice. The information in this book has been provided for educational and entertainment purposes only.

The information contained in this book has been compiled from sources deemed reliable, and it is accurate to the best of the Author's knowledge; however, the Author cannot guarantee its accuracy and validity and cannot be held liable for any errors or omissions. Changes are periodically made to this book. You must consult your doctor or get professional medical advice before using any of the suggested remedies, techniques, or information in this book.

Upon using the information contained in this book, you agree to hold harmless the Author from and against any damages, costs, and expenses, including any legal fees potentially resulting from the application of any of the information provided by this guide. This disclaimer applies to any damages or injury caused by the use and application, whether directly or indirectly, of any advice or information presented, whether for breach of contract, tort, negligence, personal injury, criminal intent, or under any other cause of action.

You agree to accept all risks of using the information presented inside this book. You need to consult a professional medical practitioner in order to ensure you are both able and healthy enough to participate in this program.

Table of Contents

INTRODUCTION 1

CHAPTER 1: WHY MAKE YOUR OWN SOAP? 2

CHAPTER 2: BEST HOMEMADE SOAP RECIPES 11

CHAPTER 3: ANTIBACTERIAL WIPES 24

Handmade Hand Sanitizing Wipes 27
Diy Antibacterial Wipes 28
Homemade Antibacterial Wipes 29
Diy Reusable Antibacterial Wipes 32
Herbal Antibacterial Wipes 34
Reusable Disinfecting Wipes 36
All Natural, Reusable Homemade Wipes 38
Diy Lysol Or Clorox Wipes 40
Make Your Own Cleaning Wipes 43
Natural Disinfecting Wipes 45

CHAPTER 4: CHOOSE YOUR WEAPON 48

CHAPTER 5: BASIC SOAP MAKING INGREDIENTS 56

CHAPTER 7: MAIN INGREDIENTS 80

CHAPTER 8: THE NITTY-GRITTIES OF HERBAL SOAP MAKING 99

CHAPTER 9: BASIC TECHNIQUES IN MAKING YOUR SOAP BAR OR LIQUID SOAP 107

CHAPTER 10: A LITTLE MORE INSIGHT INTO THE INGREDIENTS 130

CHAPTER 11: SOAP MAKING PROCESS 142

Cold Process Soaps 146
Hot Process Soaps.. 149
Re-Batching Soap 156
Making Transparent Soap... 158

CHAPTER 12: COLD PROCESS RECIPES........................... 168

CONCLUSION.. 202

Introduction

You have found the perfect business idea, and now you are ready to take the next step. There is more to starting a business than just registering it with the state. We have put together this simple guide to starting your soap making business. These steps will ensure that your new business is well planned out, registered properly and legally compliant.

Chapter 1: Why Make Your Own Soap?

Even if you can make soap safely in your own home some people will still question why you should bother doing it. After all you can buy a year's worth of soap for only a few dollars – even if you desired fancier soap most people can only go through so many bars a month.

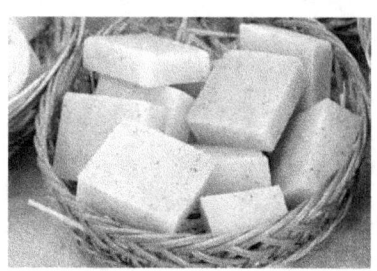

If it were indeed the case that you only wanted three smaller bars of soap for yourself then making an entire batch of soap probably would seem as unnecessary as baking a whole cake when you just wanted a slice.

But there are two good reasons for making your own soap. Firstly, you can control everything that goes into the soap when you make it. If you're allergic to anything or you don't want to have certain chemicals used on your skin, you are in control of that.

Industrially made soap can sometimes dry out your skin and may have been stripped of some of its natural moisturizing properties. Homemade soap, by contrast, is often good for people that suffer from eczema or other skin conditions and retains all of its natural moisturizing and cleaning properties.

Being able to choose the colors and scents you use is helpful as well. You can use completely natural dyes for your soap and control the scents entirely. Why use lavender extract when you can use actual lavender from your garden?

The second big advantage of homemade soap is that you can make a lot of it relatively quickly and once you have the basic ingredients and materials it can be made for not much money. There are many uses to having lots of fantastic soap at your disposal.

If you run a salon or hotel it can be a great selling point that you offer customers some of your homemade soap to use. You can sell it easily at markets or online, or even to other hotels and salons in the area.

If you happen to live in a region where a particularly nice smelling plant grows in abundance you have a potentially huge market to sell authentic soap using that plant.

Then of course you can give soap out as gifts and save yourself and your family lots of money over time with your homemade soap.

What this guide will teach you

The main purpose of this guide is to give you a step-by-step guide in making soap at home using both a hot and cold soap making process. We won't skip out any details to make sure that you know what you are doing and ensuring you are staying safe at every step of the way.

Making soap is a relatively simply process but if you don't know what you're doing then something as feeble as stirring incorrectly can be the difference between crumbly soap and wonderfully creamy soap.

We'll start by looking at what soap actually is and how it works then we'll go over the different processes in this book and which you might want to choose.

Next we'll look at the different ingredients you'll need, how to get hold of them cheaply, and go over some ideas for scents and dyes you might want to use.

Then we get to the really good part and how to make your own soap using hot and cold techniques. We'll provide you clear and detailed instructions for every step of the way and tricks for staying safe and getting the best soap possible.

What is soap?

Even though you might have been aware that soap can be dangerous to make, you, like many of us, may never have thought about how you can safely rub it all over your skin every morning.

To get the best results out of your soap it is helpful to know how soap works, what the different components do for your skin, and how the soap making process actually works.

The science isn't too important in understanding or learning how to make soap, but having a better grasp of it can help you make sense of why you are doing what you are doing.

How soap cleans your body

Soap is essentially just a type of salt that you get when you treat a fat or oil with a corrosive substance or alkali.

You should note here that 'salt' doesn't just refer to the table salt that you season your food with. A 'salt' is any compound that is created after an acid reacts with a base. In this case the acid is the fatty acid of an oil or fat (the same fatty acids that you eat) and the base (the thing that neutralizes the acid) is usually lye.

This salt can be dissolved in water and this allows it to reduce the surface tension of water so it can be spread around your skin. The soap attracts both water and the oils and soils (aka dirt) that are otherwise resistant to water. Once in this soapy state you can then blast the dirt and soap off you with water.

This leaves behind a less oily skin and hopefully a nice perfume on your skin.

Using different combinations of fats and alkalis will give you different types of soaps – the soap you use to clean your body works in the same way as the soaps used to clean dishes or cars.

The type of alkali you use will determine whether soap is very hard or whether it is soft.

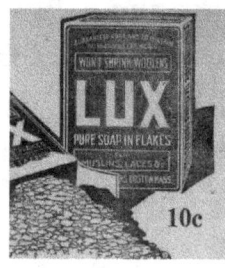

How soap is made

There are several ways to make the soap you know as soap but the underlying chemical process is very similar for each. You get a fat and you 'treat' it in some form or another with an alkaline solution. Usually this is mixing them together (as is the case with 'cold process' soap) or boiling the ingredients together and then extracting the soap away from the water.

The chemical process is called saponification. What happens during saponification is that the fatty acids of the fat become loose and then form together again as a new substance that includes fats, alkali, salts, and glycerin.

Glycerin is a scary sounding substance but it's perfectly natural and safe when made from things like animal or vegetable fat. It can then be used as a moisturizer and to exfoliate skin.

If you've read the book Fight Club (or watched the film) you might have wondered what the connection really is between soap and dynamite. Dynamite is also known as nitroglycerin and to make that you need glycerin which you can get from regular fat with the above process.

The energy you make from fat when you eat is essentially the same energy used for explosions. But don't worry, unless you intentionally nitrate your glycerin it's not dangerous.

One of the advantages of making your own soap is that the glycerin stays in (or it can be removed in some soap making processes) and you get all the health benefits of that. This is especially good for people with dry skin disorders.

What's in soap?

To make a soap that will clean you all you need is a fat, an alkali, and water. Most people choose to add a perfume and some coloring but those ingredients don't specifically help the soap be soapy.

Later we will look at the different types of fats you can use and what the story is with lye.

Chapter 2: Best Homemade Soap Recipes

Here are some of the best homemade soap recipes in the world, so let's see why they are so beautiful and special.

1. Oh, honey, honey

* Melt and pour process

If you are looking for ways to fight acnes and/or aging, this is the way to go. The combination of milk and honey is unparalleled. It will make your skin soft and nourished, while also adding anti-aging and acne-fighting properties. This is "Pour and melt" method, so you will need about 1lb of Goat's milk soap base, 3 Tbl. organic raw honey, and one drop of yellow and red soap colorants. For a real honey shape, buy a silicone honeycomb mold. When the soap is melted, add honey and colorants.

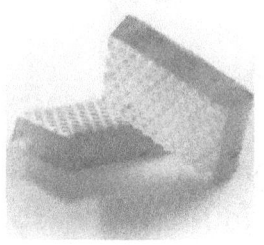

2. Do you believe in miracles? – Aloe Vera Soap

* Cold process

Aloe Vera is well known for its healthy properties, from soothing burns and cuts to anti-inflammatory properties, to soothing muscles, healing wounds and bruises, so you just have to take the advantage of it.

You need 7.5 oz mineral water, 0.4 oz beeswax, 3 oz lye, 1.5 lbs olive oil, 1.8 oz Aloe Vera juice, and 0.18 oz mint essential oil. Use a large saucepan for mixing lye into the water and stir until dissolved. The temperature needs to be 130 degrees F. In another saucepan, heat olive oil to 130 degrees F and stir in beeswax carefully. Remove the oil mixture from the oven and add the lye mixture to it. Stir every 15 minutes until you get a consistent texture. Add aloe Vera juice and essential oil and stir for one minute. Then pour the mixture into molds and follow the basic steps that I mentioned above.

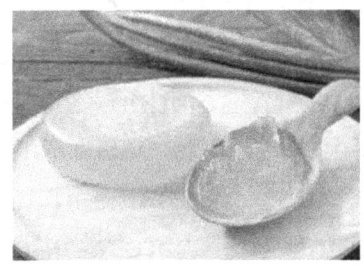

3. Black Magic

* Cold process

If you have oily skin, this black soap is perfect for you. With tea tree oil and activated charcoal, this soap will do wonders to your skin. Add to that coconut, palm, Tamanu and castor oils and you get deeply moisturizing and refreshing soap.

You need 5.1 oz. Sodium Hydroxide Lye, 10.1 oz. Distilled Water, 2 Tbsp. Activated Charcoal, 1.8 oz. Castor Oil (5%), 14.4 oz. Olive Oil (40%), 9 oz. Coconut Oil (25%),1.8 oz. Tamanu Oil (5%), 9 oz. Palm Oil (25%) and 1.7 oz. Tea Tree Essential Oil and 12 bar rectangle silicone molds. After you have made the lye solution set it aside to cool. In another bowl completely melt oils (but not essential oil) and leave it to cool a bit. When both solutions have reached 110 degrees, add the lye solution to the oils. Then add charcoal and use a stick blender to mix the charcoal into the soap. Just remember to put a stick blender into the mixture first and then to turn it on. Next, add tea tree essential oil and repeat the process with the stick blender. After that, follow the basic steps to pour the mixture into molds. Spritz the top of your soap with alcohol in order to prevent soda ash.

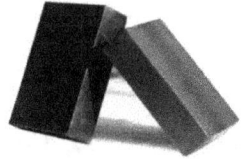

4. Purple Rain

* Melt and pour process

If you have sensitive and dry skin, you will love this simple Lavender Oatmeal soap recipe. While Lavender has a calming effect on you and your skin, it is also great for skin detoxification and improving circulation. Oats, on the other hand, help soothe dry and sensitive skin, while removing dead skin cells and cleaning the skin.

You need 9-10 oz. goat's milk soap, ¼ cup quick cook oats, 1 tbs lavender flowers (dried) and ¼ tsp lavender essential oil. This recipe is a breeze to make, yet it delivers so many benefits. Just follow the above pour and melt method and you'll be fine.

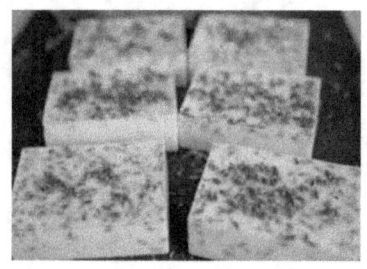

5. Make every soap count

This recipe is all about turning those scraps of soap bars into new ones with a simple method. Use as many soap scraps as you can and cut them into small pieces. Then place them into a pot and add enough water to cover the soap bars. Cook at the medium temperature and let it simmer for a couple of minutes. Keep in mind that you have to stir often so that the mixture gets consistent. Put a pan under a steel colander so as to preserve the soap drippings and make use of them. With a wooden spoon drain the excess water out of soap until you get a nice texture. Then, pour the mixture into molds or glass bowls and let it cool.

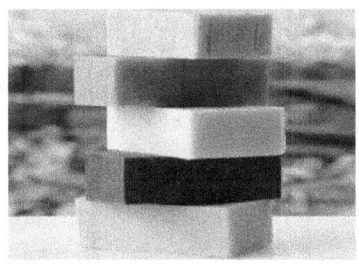

6. Brighten your day

*Cold process

The Calendula soap is ideal for protecting and hydrating your skin, leaving it soft and smooth. Moreover, this soap contains high-quality oils that only add up to the beauty of your skin. This soap also makes a great gift because it looks striking.

You need 226 g lye, 500 g distilled water, 500 g olive oil, 470 g coconut oil, 650 g rice bran oil and 16 g dried calendula petals.

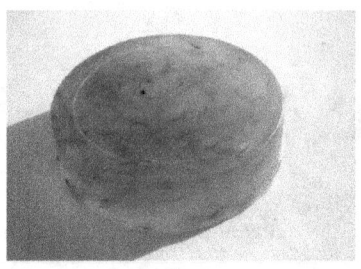

7. Smooth and lovely

*Cold process

This recipe is a real treat for your skin, due to all the oils and Shea butter. You can add essential oil of your choice if you want. Shea butter has anti-inflammatory properties and is a great antioxidant. Jojoba oil is great for controlling oily skin and acne, while the avocado oil is a natural sunblock and protects skin from damage. Coconut oil smells sensational and other oils also contribute to making your skin shiny and healthy.

You need 4 oz. Avocado Oil, 1 oz. Jojoba Oil, 8 oz. Coconut Oil, 16 oz. Olive Oil, 4 oz. Shea Butter, 8 oz. Palm Oil, 5.6 oz. Lye and 11 – 15 oz. Water.

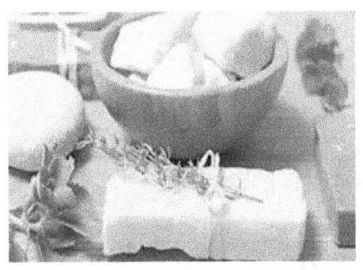

8. A nourishing bomb

*Cold process

This soap is ideal for winter when your skin is dry and needs oils to bring it back to life. Thanks to Hemp seed oil, your tired skin will be rejuvenated while Shea butter will make it soft again. Sweet Almond Oil, Avocado Oil, Coconut and Palm oil will give your skin just what it needs to cope with the freezing challenges of winter.

You need 2 oz. Sweet Almond Oil, 8 oz. Coconut Oil, 2 oz. Avocado Oil, 2 oz. Hempseed Oil, 8 oz. Palm Oil, 16 oz. Olive Oil, 4 oz. Shea Butter, 2 oz. Vitamin E, 2 oz. Wheatgerm Oil, 12-16 oz. Water and 6.0 oz. Lye.

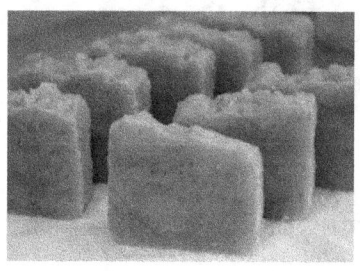

9. Marvelous combination!

* Melt and pour process

Here we have pink Himalayan Salt and Grapefruit Soap – the extraordinary combination that your skin will be thankful for. Each time you treat it with this wonderful soap, it will make your skin soft and hydrated, due to the properties of these ingredients.

You need 1 pound goat's milk soap base, 10-15 drops Grapefruit essential oil, and 1/4 cup Pink Himalayan Salt.

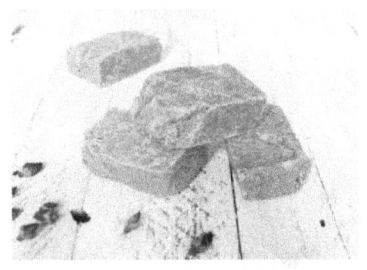

10. It's time for gifts!

* Melt and pour process

This soap recipe combines calming effects of lavender and lemon scent, leaving you energized and de-stressed. And in this crazy time we live in, everything that helps with reducing stress is welcomed, especially when it also nourishes our skin. Whether you want to surprise your mother with this gift or to spoil yourself with a unique bath experience, this is the perfect recipe for that.

You need 2 pounds Goats Milk Soap Base, 10-15 drops lavender essential oil, a few drops of purple soap dye, 10 drops lemon essential oil.

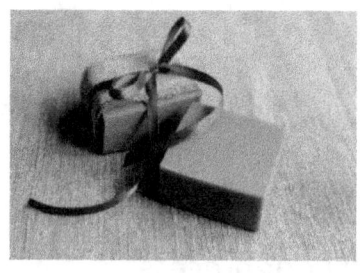

11. It gets hot!

*Hot process

If you feel skilled enough to try out this hot process soap recipe, then be my guest. Olive oil has been used for centuries for skin, and we can see why that is so. It doesn't clog pores but protects and hydrates skin. Coconut oil is a deep cleanser and helps reduce fine wrinkles on your face. Essential oil will add a nice scent to this combination.

You need 10 oz olive oil, 9 oz distilled water, 20 oz coconut oil, 4.78 oz. lye, and Essential oil of your choice. Just keep in mind that you need to add the coconut oil first so it melts completely. After that, add the olive oil and follow other steps for hot process soapmaking.

Chapter 3: Antibacterial Wipes

In regards to keeping yourself, your body and your home clean, antibacterial and disinfecting wipes are going to play an important role. Wipes can be used to disinfect surfaces like tables, countertops, and commonly touched points. Touchpoints include doorknobs, handles on refrigerators and appliances, car steering wheels, and any other surface that is touched by different people throughout the day. After unloading your groceries, use your DIY antibacterial wipes to clean off your countertops so they are safe the next time you begin to prepare food.

Wipes can be used to clean off your hands or a child's hands if something sticky or dirty is touched or picked up. You can also use homemade wipes for changing baby's diapers. Be sure you dispose of them properly after you use them.

Wipes are handy too: you can keep them in a glove compartment, or even in a purse or backpack. Wipes are great, but they can get pricey when used regularly. Making your own wipes has a few different benefits. First and foremost, it can be less expensive. The materials you use to make these wipes often come in quantities that can be used for multiple batches. Another benefit is that you can also make reusable wipes so that you produce less waste and have a positive impact on the environment.

Reusable wipes reduce your waste impact, but they do require a little more maintenance. After using them, they do need to be properly laundered before they can be used again. In some cases, you can reuse your wipes several times, returning them to their container and the sanitization liquid inside to clean them.

After a while, it is still recommended that you launder these wipes and refresh the sanitizing solution. Use your discretion on how you want to make the most out of your reusable wipes, and consider what you've used them on and how soiled the wipe is.

Furthermore, some commercial wipes can contain irritating chemicals and substances that cause the skin or break out or to dry out. Many of the provided recipes offer natural solutions to wipes that are just as effective but don't have the same topical impact. The provided instructions are safe for adults and children, however, if you or a child experiences skin irritation from using the wipes, it is best to talk to a medical professional and try a different solution.

It is important to store your wipes properly so they remain moist. If they dry out they are no longer effective as an antibacterial cleaning option.

Handmade Hand Sanitizing Wipes

Materials and Tools

- ¼ cup hot water

- 2 tbsp aloe vera gel

- 1½ cup 99% rubbing alcohol

- Dry, unscented wipes such as body wipes or baby wipes

- Container with lid (glass or plastic Tupperware, or a ziplock bag for easy storage)

- A mixing bowl and spoon

<u>Instructions</u>

Put your wipes in your Tupperware container or in your ziplock bag.

In your mixing bowl, combine the water, aloe, and rubbing alcohol together. Use the spoon to blend the ingredients together until you get a smooth mixture.

Pour the solution over your wipes and let them soak until they are saturated, then you can pour away the excess. If you're using dry wipes, you might need to double up on the recipe amounts to ensure full saturation.

If you don't use the wipes fast enough, they might dry out. If they do begin to dry out, you can re-dampen them with the same solution to continue using the wipes.

Diy Antibacterial Wipes

Materials and Tools

- 2 cups warm distilled water

- 1 cup 70% or higher isopropyl alcohol

- 1 tbsp dish soap

- 10 drops thieves essential oil (or another disinfecting essential oil)

- Roll of paper towels

● Sealable glass container that can hold the paper towel roll

● Glass pitcher or measuring cup

Instructions

Set your paper towels in the sealable glass container.

In your pitcher, mix the alcohol, distilled water, essential oil, and dish soap together. Mix gently to avoid excess bubbles and blend together thoroughly.

Pour your solution over the paper towels and seal the container. Let the paper towels soak for 30 minutes before pouring away the excess solution.

These wipes are great for disinfecting surfaces.

Homemade Antibacterial Wipes
Materials and Tools

- 1 cup of homemade or natural scent-free lotion

- 1 cup rubbing alcohol of at least 70%

- 15 drops of disinfectant or antibacterial essential oil, such as tea tree or lemon

- Heavy-duty paper towels

- Sealable plastic or glass container

- Ziplock bags

- Scissors

Instructions

Add the rubbing alcohol, lotion, and essential oil to one of your ziplock bags. Make sure to seal it close and expel as much air as possible.

Knead the bag carefully so you don't break the seams and the ingredients don't spill out. Keep kneading until the solution is well mixed.

Cut your paper towels into halves or thirds. A whole paper towel is likely going to be too big for single-use wipes. Cutting the paper will also yield you more wipes.

Put your paper towels in the sealable container and then pour your solution mixture onto the towels. If you have too many towel pieces to fit in the container, break up the rest into stacks that will fit inside ziplock bags for portability. Mix up another batch of the solution and use half of it per small batch of wipes.

Once all the wipes are covered, let them soak for at least 30 minutes in the solution. Every 10 minutes, flip the container or bags upside down to keep the solution moving through the stacks of wipes.

Pour away the excess solution. The lotion in these wipes can help keep the skin moisturized which makes them a good option for baby wipes. Double-check on your chosen essential oil to ensure that it is suitable for use with infants and small children. If the wipes are meant specifically for children, you might want to reduce the essential oil to 10 drops instead of 15.

Diy Reusable Antibacterial Wipes

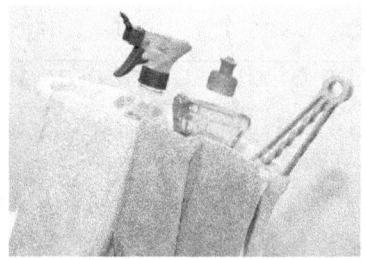

Materials and Tools

- 70% or higher rubbing alcohol

- Liquid castile soap (like Dr. Bronner's)

- Tea tree essential oil (optional)

- Lavender essential oil (optional)

- Warm distilled or filtered water

- 1 or 2-ply flannel baby wipes, unscented (8 in by 8 in)

- Empty baby wipes container

- Mixing bowl

<u>Instructions</u>

Mix warm filtered or distilled water with 1 tablespoon of your castile soap. Add in ½ cup of rubbing alcohol and mix until all the ingredients are combined.

If you're using essential oils, add in three to five drops of each and mix them in.

Fold your flannel wipes one on top of the other, and tuck them into the wipe containers, then pour your antibacterial solution over them.

Let the wipes saturate for at least 30 minutes before use.

Keep the container closed to prevent them from drying out.

When the wipes get used or soiled, launder them and then re-saturate them with the same solution to turn them back into fresh wipes for reuse.

Herbal Antibacterial Wipes

Materials and Tools

- ¼ cup isopropyl alcohol, 99%
- 1 tsp lavender oil
- 1 tsp tea tree oil
- 1 tsp eucalyptus oil
- ½ tsp clove essential oil
- ½ tsp rosemary oil
- 15 heavy-duty paper towels
- Scissors
- Sealable glass or plastic jar with a lid

- Measure cup or mixing bowl

Instructions

Begin by ripping your paper towels apart on the perforated line and cutting each towel into quarters.

Next, roll the towels up into one big roll. Begin rolling one piece into a snug roll. Tuck the end of the next piece into the roll and roll that towel section around the originally rolled towel. Continue this process until all the towels are rolled together into a large roll. Tucking them into each other this way will make it so that when you pull one towel out, another towel will be moved into position to take its place.

Put your wipe roll into your jar. They should fit snugly in the round container.

In a large glass measuring cup or in a mixing bowl, mix the alcohol and the essential oils. Make sure to blend the ingredients well.

Slowly pour the combined antibacterial mixture over your rolled paper towels in the jar. Close the lid and let them soak until saturated, at least 30 minutes. You can either leave the wipes in the mixture or pour out any excess liquid.

When you use the wipes, pull out the outermost wipe up from inside the jar. Since the wipes are tucked together, this will pull the next wipe up so you can access it easier the next time you pull one out.

Reusable Disinfecting Wipes

Materials and Tools

- 1 cup cooled distilled or filtered water

- 1 cup white vinegar

- 2 teaspoons fragrance-free, biodegradable detergent

- 12 drops lavender essential oil

- 5 drops of any essential oil, such as grapefruit, lemon, or tea tree

- Microfiber cloths, 8 in by 8 in

- Airtight plastic or glass container with a lid

- Label

- Jug or jar for mixing

- Jar for saturation

<u>Instructions</u>

Fold your wipes in half, stacking them on top of each other, then put the stack into one of the jars. This is where your wipes are going to soak up the disinfectant solution.

In the other jar or jug, combine water, detergent, essential oils, vinegar, and water. Mix with a spoon, or if the jar has a lid, close the lid and swish around until well combined.

Pour the liquid over the wipes in the saturation jar. Seal the jar and let the cloths soak for at least 30 minutes to completely saturate them.

Pour off the excess liquid and move the microfiber cloths to your sealable white or plastic container. Put a label on the container to ensure everybody knows what it contains.

When the wipes get used or soiled, launder them and soak them again in the same solution to turn them back into disinfectant wipes.

All Natural, Reusable Homemade Wipes

Materials and Tools

- 2 cups distilled or filtered water

- 1 cup rubbing alcohol, at least 70%

- 5 drops tea tree oil

- 5 drops lavender oil

- 5 drops thyme oil

- 5 drops cinnamon oil

- Terrycloth washcloths

- Quart size mason jar with lid

Instructions

Start by pouring water and rubbing alcohol into your mason far, and stir until well combined.

Next, add in your essential oils. Be mindful of how many drops you are adding, and don't add too many or the concentration will be too potent. Use a spoon to mix the oils into the alcohol and water, or put the mason jar lid on securely and shake the jar until all ingredients are combined.

Roll your terrycloth washcloths into individual rolls and place them in the mason jar, sticking one end right into the essential oil mixture. Put as many towel rolls into the jar as can comfortably fit without excess squishing.

Let the cloths soak up the liquid solution for at least 30 minutes before use. Leave them in the sealed jar for freshness.

When your clothes have been used, launder them and then mix up a new batch of the essential oil disinfectant to use them again and again.

Diy Lysol Or Clorox Wipes

Materials and Tools

- 2 ¼ cup ethanol alcohol

- 2 tablespoons hydrogen peroxide

- 15 drops lemon essential oil

- 15 drops tea tree essential oil

- ½ cup distilled or filtered water

- Roll of paper towels

- Non-serrated knife

- A sealable jar that can hold ½ roll of paper towels

- Glass measuring cup, pitcher, or mixing bowl

Instructions

Your first step is going to be cutting your paper towel roll in half. Use a non-serrated knife so that you don't tear the paper towels to shreds. Be careful when cutting the roll and make sure the knife is sharp enough to accomplish the task.

Set one half of the paper towel roll inside your selected jar.

In your mixing receptacle of choice, add all the liquid ingredients and the essential oils. Mix them together thoroughly and then pour over the paper towels.

Let the roll saturate for 30 minutes minimum, then carefully remove the cardboard roll from the center of the paper towels. This will pull up the center towel for easy access. As you remove wipes from the roll, another one will be pulled up to take its place. You can pour off any excess liquid if you would like.

If you have two jars that can hold half a paper towel roll, double up on the ingredient measurements and turn both paper towel roll halves into a set of disinfecting wipes.

For your second roll, try different essential oil combinations with some other options such as eucalyptus, thyme, cinnamon, clove, rosemary, chamomile, orange, lavender, or peppermint oils. You can use two to three oils, adjusting the quantities to get 30 to 45 drops of oil total.

Make Your Own Cleaning Wipes

Materials and Tools

- ½ cup vinegar

- ¼ cup distilled or filtered water

- ¼ cup rubbing alcohol, at least 70%

- 1 teaspoon liquid dish soap

- 1 pound coffee canister with lid, empty of coffee grounds and cleaned out

- Sharp knife

- Paper towel roll

- Needle

- Scissors

- Spray paint (optional)

- Mixing bowl or pitcher

Instructions

If you'd like to hide the coffee logo and design on your can, take the optional step of spray painting your can and can lid before you get started. Once the paint is dry, proceed to step two. If you aren't painting your can, start with step two.

Cut your paper towel roll in half with a sharp, non-serrated knife. Press half of the paper towel roll into the coffee can.

In your bowl or pitcher, mix together the vinegar, water, rubbing alcohol and dish soap. Mix carefully so that you don't get a lot of soap bubbles.

Slowly drizzle the antibacterial mixture over the paper towels in the coffee can.

Let the paper towels sit and soak up the liquid for at least 30 minutes and then gently remove the cardboard roll from the center. The central towel will be pulled up from the middle of the roll. This is going to be the towel that you pull from, a new one taking its place when you rip one off.

Using your needle, poke several small holes into the center of the coffee can lid, then use your scissors to poke the holes out until they are all connecting. This is going to be the hole you pull your wipes from. You want your hole to be about ½ inch in diameter.

Carefully pull the lifted towel through the hole in the coffee can lid partway, and then snap the lid in place.

Keep in mind that the wipe sticking out of the top of the can might dry out if it isn't used fast enough. If that happens pull the top wipe out and use the next one.

Natural Disinfecting Wipes

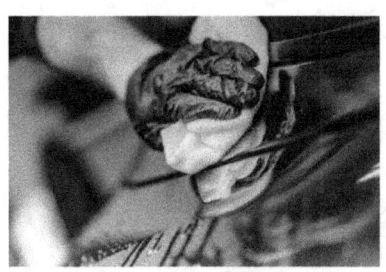

Materials and Tools

- ¾ cup distilled white vinegar

- ¾ cup distilled or filtered water

- 15 drops lemon essential oil

- 4 drops bergamot essential oil

- 8 drops lavender essential oil

- Wide mouth, quart-sized mason jar with lid

- 15-20 precut cloth rags, like from old cotton t-shirts

Instructions

Pour the water and vinegar into your mason jar. Mix them with a spoon. Once they are combined, add the essential oils.

Using a spoon, mix the oils into the vinegar and water combination.

Fold your precut clothes so that they will fit comfortably inside your mason jar.

Put the cloths in the jar and press them down so that each cloth touches the liquid, then secure the lid.

Turn the jar upside down and set on a flat surface, allowing at least 30 minutes for the cloths to soak up the liquid before using them.

Once you use a wipe, or when it gets too dirty, launder the cloths and make a fresh batch of the disinfectant solution to soak them in for another round of wipes.

Chapter 4: Choose Your Weapon

All the Tools That You Need

In this chapter I will go through the equipment that you are going to need to help you make your own soaps. A big advantage when it comes to soap crafting is that there is not a wide range of specialized equipment needed. In fact, a lot of the items that you need you will most likely already have and the rest can easily be picked up inexpensively.

That said, you will need a separate set of tools for soap making – you cannot, for example, use a bowl for mixing soap batter and then use it for making cake batter, no matter how well you wash it out. Soap making involves the use of lye and lye, if ingested, can be toxic and burn. It is much better not to take any chances in this regard.

When it comes to containers, stainless steel, hard plastic and glass are your only options. Metals such as brass, aluminum and bronze or out of the question as these will react with the lye to dangerous effect.

Your Basic Basics

Here is a list of the basic basics:

Plastic wrap or freezer paper to use to protect your work area and to line metal molds, if necessary.

A knife, non-serrated, to cut bars of soap with.

A rack to cure your soap on – this requires ventilation on all sides of the bar.

Droppers for adding colors or essential oil blends.

A spatula made of silicon.

Spoons for stirring – stainless steel are your best bet, Teflon reacts with the lye and wood will be corroded by the lye.

A whisk – either silicon or stainless steel.

Glass or stainless steel bowls.

Glass measuring jug and a set of stainless steel measuring cups to get the amount of ingredients right.

Two candy thermometers made of glass or stainless steel. (If you can only get one, that's fine but two makes life a lot easier.)

A double boiler (alternatively, make your own using one pot in a bigger one.)

A slow-cooker (not strictly necessary).

A microwave.

A hand-held immersion blender. (These are not expensive to find at the store and save you so much effort when it comes to tracing the soap that they are an absolute essential item.) You just need an entry-level blender that has smooth bottom edge. You don't need to find one with a lot of speed settings either. A blender can cut the time it takes to trace by something like 90% - well worth it, don't you think. (Ask someone who used to stand stirring the soap manually for 45 minutes until it traced.)

An accurate scale is essential and I advise spending a little more on an electronic scale that can handle higher weights. In a lot of cases, you will need to use the glass/stainless steel container that your ingredients will be poured into when it comes to weighing them.

A soap mold can be made out of just about anything as long as it can stand up to the heat. I have even used a cardboard milk carton lined with freezer paper in a pinch. You can get specialized molds for soap making that allow you to pour blocks of soap that you can cut later and these are very handy if you are going to be making a lot of soap. As long as the mold is sturdy enough to hold the weight of the poured soap and can withstand the heat, you can use just about anything. All you need to do is to ensure that it is fully lined with freezer paper, dull side facing the mold, before pouring your soap. Containers that you are able to flex will make it easier to release your soap so steer clear of glass.

Make Your Own Miter Box for Soap Pouring

You will need a hand-held saw, 10 x 1 inch screws, a screwdriver, wood strips measuring 4 inches wide, half an inch thick and twice as long as the miter box plus an extra eight inches. You will also need a 2 inch strip that is the same length as the strip above. A pre-made miter box and a drill round out your supplies.

From the half inch thick wood, cut two lengths that are equal in length to the miter box.

From the 1 inch thick wood, cut two lengths that are equal in length to the miter box.

Mark out three evenly-spaced marks on the 1 inch strips and drill through these. Continue in the same manner with the half inch strips but not all the way through this time.

Screw the different strips together and place into the miter box.

Measure the opening between each of the sides. Your end pieces will be cute from this and must fit securely so that the soap does not leak out at all.

Cut the remaining pieces of 1 inch wood so that the will close off the ends of the box and fit snugly.

You can now adjust the size of the bar by moving the ends of the box in or out, as you require.

Alternatively, you can also use a piece of PVC piping to mold your soaps in, just be sure to rub the inside with petroleum jelly and closing off one end securely before pouring your soap into it.

When in doubt about whether an object can be used as a soap mold or not, to see if can be put in the microwave or dishwasher. If it can be, this usually means that it will work as a mold as well.

If you have a container that you want to use but are not sure whether it will be big enough for your recipe, simply fill it with water and measure how much water it can contain. Convert that to cubic inches by multiplying it by 1.8. 40% of this measurement will give you the amount of fat your soap will need to contain to fill out the container. Then work out the lye content, etc. based on that fat total.

Make Your Own Curing Stands

You will also need a rack to lay your soap one while it is drying. For small batches, a stainless steel dish rack or baking rack is fine. If you are going to make larger batches, it is simple enough to make your own curing rack – Simply get four plain pieces of lumber to make a frame and staple a layer of plastic mesh over it. I have three such racks that I can layer when I need to – I simply put a couple of bricks between each layer to separate them out and find that this makes storing the soap while it is curing a whole lot easier.

Chapter 5: Basic Soap Making Ingredients

The most basic ingredients of soap are base oil and lye. There are other things that are added along the way to make the soap smell good, lather gently and look beautiful. Here are some of the basic ingredients of Soap.

Base Oils

Base Oils also called heavy Oils, are produced by refining crude oil. Once the crude oil is heated, various distillates are separated from one another, making heavy oils suitable for base oils. These oils can be animal based or vegetable based. However, vegetable oils are preferred because they have better benefits than animal fat. Animal fat takes too long to process and may have a foul smell.

Basic soap recipes should be in proportions of 30 % coconut oil, 40 % olive oil, and 30% palm oil. Depending on the type of soap you want to make while creating a new recipe you can replace some or all of one or more of these with some special oils that has similar qualities.

The most basic base oils used in soap making are:

- Olive Oil

Olive oil is probably the oldest and most popular base oil in the soap making processes. Olive oil is good if you intend to make exfoliating soaps. It is proven to help exfoliate dead skin cells and gives you smoother and younger-looking skin. It also helps unclog pores. It is also very good for newborns with skin issues, and it is rich in antioxidants and vitamin E. Besides for the skin, it is very good for the hair as well. Therefore, it is also very often used for making shampoo. Olive oil is soft/hard oil because it makes very soft soap in the beginning, but cures into a very hard soap bar. The lather is rather slippery with almost no bubbles; therefore, it is recommended to combine this oil with other base oils. Soap with 50% or more of olive oil is called Castile soap.

- Coconut Oil

Coconut oil is a great moisturizer. It keeps the skin hydrated, and it is recommended for dry skin. It helps soothe and nourish the skin and eliminates a flaky appearance. It also helps minimize the skin pores, making the skin look smoother. Coconut Oil has a high level of lauric acid which gives it a great effect as an antibacterial. Its lather is very rich and high cleansing.

- Palm Oil

Palm oil has a natural glycerin, beta carotene, and vitamin E. It is recommended for sensitive skin. Because of its antioxidants, it keeps the skin younger looking and protected from dirt and radicals that may cause irritations. Despite the high level of cleansing, it is recommended to combine with other base oils for its nutrition value is rather low.

Special Oils

Special oils are lighter oils than the base oils. They are usually added to the base oil to address specific skin issues. A base oil may also be used as a special oil.

Special oils usually take up 10% of the oils needed for the recipe. They cannot be made into base oils because they are lighter and may make the soap soft. Also, some of them may have an adverse effect on the skin if a large amount is used.

Below are some of the most common special oils added to soap:

- Shea Butter. This butter is an ivory-colored famous moisturizer full of vitamin A. It is added to almost all cosmetic products. It prevents drying and chapping of the skin and is known to soothe insect bites or sunburns. Shea butter is hard oil with mild, lotion- like lather.

- Cocoa Butter. This also acts as a moisturizer. Cocoa butter is famous for its mild fragrance and ultra-hydrating. Unlike the Shea butter, it has more antioxidants and can help eradicate dark spots.

- Mango Butter. This product is relatively new to the cosmetic industry, but it has been proven to be great for the skin. It is a good moisturizer and antioxidant. It can also help whiten the skin and helps eliminate wrinkles and other skin blemishes. Mango butter also protects your skin from sunburn or can sooth already sunburned skin.

• Avocado Oil. Aside from being a moisturizer, this oil helps in the regeneration of cells. It helps in maintaining the suppleness of the skin, and it tightens the pores, making the skin smoother. Avocado oil has a high amount of omega 3 fatty acids and proteins which are highly beneficial for the skin and hair.

• Sweet Almond Oil. If you desire to make a gentle soap for babies or younger children, you should add this oil. Sweet almond oil will make your soap hypoallergenic. It is a great addition to soaps for people with sensitive skin. It also helps treat skin rashes and eczema in children.

• Castor Oil. This is a good oil for making antimicrobial soaps. It helps treat skin diseases and eliminate scars and blemishes. It also controls acne breakouts and can help prevent wrinkles and tighten the skin, minimizing the appearance of pores. Precautions should be given when you use castor oil. It is known to induce labor in pregnant women. It may not have the same effects when applied on the skin, but precautions should still be taken.

- Jojoba oil. This oil applies to all skin types. It helps moisturize dry skin and controls the production of oil. It is safe to add to baby soaps. A very important thing about this oil is that it has replaced animal fats in many skin lotions and other beauty products.

- Aloe Vera oil. This oil helps with the cell regeneration of the skin, making the skin look younger. However, Aloe Vera can make the skin oily. It is not recommended for use by those with oily skin or sensitive skin. Aloe Vera contains vitamins C, E, B as well as minerals, proteins, amino acids, and beta-carotene.

- Peanut oil has a very good cleaning effect on your skin and a lather that is perfect for soft soaps. It is highly nutritious for your skin.

- Apricot Kernel oil, as well as Sunflower oil, are soft oils that provide medium lather and mild cleansing. It is a great addition to the olive oil in a recipe.

There are three types of base oils- hard, brittle and soft. Soaps with a higher percentage of hard and brittle oils harden much faster. If you are using a high percentage of soft oils in your soap- it might take those a couple extra days to cure. Soaps with soft oils are much easier for swirling and coloring.

Lye

A couple of hundred years ago, making a good batch of soap was more an art than a science and just as there were famous people for their cooking, some were well known and appreciated for their art of soap making. The difficulties of soap making mostly concerned the lye.

Measuring the lye, long before digital scales, was the main problem. Most of the soap making attempts ended up with either too harsh or too soft to use soaps.

Today, lye can easily be measured by using a digital scale which will be one of your best friends in the soap making processes.

Lye is the chemical that turns the oil into soap. There are two kinds of lye that are used in soap making. These are the sodium hydroxide and the potassium hydroxide.

The sodium hydroxide is added when you want to make hard soaps. Potassium hydroxide is added when you want to make liquid soaps. If you want to make a creamy soap, you will need to combine specific amounts of the two types of lye.

One thing you must pay great attention to is dealing with the safety risk when working with lye. Therefore, it is very important, once you decide to use the soap making process with lye, to clear your schedule and be fully dedicated to the process while handling the lye.

In making lye solutions, always pour the lye into the liquid. The water may fizzle more if it is poured over the lye solution and may cause an accident in your kitchen.

Water

Water is needed for making the lye solution. Water is very important to dissolve the lye and for the hydrolysis to the fat. Too much water will produce too soft soap bars.

Distilled water or clean spring water is preferred. Tap water may have chemicals that can cause other reactions with the lye.

Essential Oils

Essential oils are not necessary for soap making. They are often added for the purpose of adding fragrance to the soap. However, there are other essential oils that make the soap healthier. Some essential oils are also added to make specific soaps for a particular skin type or problem. Essential oils are also believed to have a powerful therapeutic effect. Just one drop of essential oils can have powerful health benefits so make sure to choose your essential oils wisely.

Here are some of the most helpful essential oils that can be used for your soaps:

• Geranium oil. This oil addresses almost all skin problems. It is an antimicrobial oil that helps eliminate fungus, pimples, blackheads and other skin blemishes. It also tightens the pores, helps prevent the formation of wrinkles and improves the skin's elasticity.

• Frankincense oil. This oil encourages cell growth, which helps in maintaining your youthful looking skin. It also protects acne-prone skin. It works as a toner and tightens the pores, making them less visible.

- Carrot Seed oil. If you want to make an anti-aging soap, you may combine this oil with palm oil. It has a lot of beta carotene and phytochemicals that help in cell regeneration. It will help a lot in making your skin look supple.

- Lavender oil. Though it is usually added as a fragrance oil, lavender can be a good essential oil in making baby soap. It can help your baby relax during and after taking a bath.

- Chamomile oil. This is another essential oil that helps you relax. It is often used for bubble bath soaps and often added to the lavender oil to stimulate the relaxing effect of the soap.

- Myrrh oil. This is a good addition to making baby soap. Myrrh is an anti-itch oil.

It helps treat skin eczema in children. It also improves the skin's elasticity.

- Rose Essential Oil. This is one of the most common yet one of the most expensive essential oils. It has a great effect on skin by lessening the stress in skin, making it healthier. It helps with water absorption and keeps the skin hydrated. It also heals cuts and wounds and other skin infections.

However, you may need a lot of oil to bring out the health benefits. Because it is expensive, it is usually only added as a fragrance oil.

- Peppermint Essential Oil. Adding some of the peppermint essential oil in your soap can provide great benefit for your skin. It is known for the ability to alleviate pain, balance hormones and heal several skin conditions. Peppermint essential oil will help relax your body.

Other Ingredients

- Dyes. If you want to add color to your soap, you should add this ingredient. The most common dye used in soap made at home is the mica powder. Food colorings may also be used. Just make sure that the dye is safe for your skin.

To make your soap entirely natural, you can use some of the natural colorants to add color to your soap. Use **grated red pepper** for apricot, red light color; **cinnamon** is great if you like your soap in light salmon color, n**ettle and mint** should be used if you would like your soap to be green; **cacao** will make your soap brown; **red cabbage** can be used for red; **indigo plant** will turn your soap into blue and **carrot** will make it orange.

- Oats, nuts, and other grains. Grains are mixed into the soap to give it a loofah-like texture. They are also good skin exfoliants.

- Honey. This makes the soap hypoallergenic. When you add honey to your soap, it is recommended that you replace some of the base oils with sweet almond oil. Honey also stimulates the antimicrobial and moisturizing effects of some of the oils.

- Natural beverages. Coffee, milk and fruit juices may also be added to add extra nutrients.

- Fruit and vegetable purees or pulps. These are mixed in to add more nutrients to the soap. If you decide to add fruits or vegetables in your soap, you will have to blend them into a watery puree and combine with water. Fruit and vegetables contain a significant amount of water and sugar so you should always dilute liquid with water to help buffer against effects of lye. Some fruits and vegetables may cause the soap to deteriorate faster, so choose those that last longer.

- Herbs, flowers, and spices. When these are mixed into the soap, their natural oil incorporates with the oil in soaps. They may also enhance the fragrance or stimulate the effectiveness of the oil in the soap. Some of the spices you can use are listed below:

- Basil. The green plant which can be added to your soap easily. You can add it either dry or simply chop the fresh basil. Once you put basil in your soap mixture, it will, most likely, turn into a dark green color. Basil is known for its relaxing and antibacterial characteristics.

- Cardamom. Asian spice which has a very nice and fresh smell. Granted cardamom improves your blood circulation and is known as a very effective energizer.

- Cinnamon. One of the most used and most popular spices in soaps. Using cinnamon in your soap will cause your soap to turn into golden brown color and will have a very relaxing effect on your skin. This is a great spice for antibacterial soap and can be used to heal some infections.

- Clove. Very strong and therapeutic smell. This spice will give your soap a brown color. It has very strong antimicrobial and antibacterial properties. Therefore, it is very often used to heal itching skin diseases such as ringworm, fungal infections, and it is considered to even kill parasites.

- Rosemary. This spice will turn your soap into a moss-like color. It is believed to have the relaxing and therapeutic effect that can even help in strengthening blood vessels or improve your memory.

How to Make Your Own Soap Recipe

Once you are familiar with all the steps in the soap making process, have tried them, and decided which one is the best for you, maybe it is time to make your own recipe for the soap.

First, you should decide which process you will use to make your soap. You can decide this based on which one you find easier and more fun for you.

It is important that you already understand all the ingredients and safety steps necessary for soap making.

For the next step, you should decide which base and (optional) essential oils, as well as the other possible ingredients you would like to use making the soap. You should have a clear picture of what you would like from your soap. From nutrition value, the level of cleansing and hardness, to the basic performance of lather and smell, everything is important to be decided in advance so you can make sure you have all the ingredients.

As we've already mentioned, handling lye is one of the most difficult things involved in the soap making process so once you decided which oils and how much of every oil you want to use, it is time to measure exactly how much of the lye and water you will need to use. Remember, even a small mistake in lye- water measuring can cause your soap to become useless.

For the simple measuring, you can use one of the online calculators. This can be handy and helpful.

In case you are an "I can do it myself" type of person, here is how you will be sure never to mistake in measuring your lye and water.

The amount of lye is calculated when you multiply the amount of fat you are going to use with a saponification value of the fat. So, the basic equation will look like this:

(Amount of fat) x (Saponification value of the fat) = (Amount of lye)

Once you have calculated the exact amount of lye you should use, divide the result with 0.3, and you will get the total weight of the lye-water solution. Equation:

(amount of lye): 0,3 = (weight of lye-water solution).

The next step is used for calculating the total amount of water that should be used in the process. You will have to subtract the amount of lye you got in the first equation from the total weight of the lye-water solution.

Equation:

(total weight of lye-water solution) - (amount of lye) = amount of water.

In case you have some extra oils that are leftover and not bounded to the lye, you may want to think about measuring the super fatting level in your soap recipe if you want to add them to your soap mixture.

You can measure this level also by using an online calculator, or you can do it all by yourself by subtracting the percentage of the super fatting level from the amount of lye. The result you get is the amount of lye that should be used in the recipe. Super fatting level should not be less than 5% and not higher than 10%. Too low super fatting percentage can cause too strong of a soap, while very high percentage can make it too greasy.

Once you make correct calculations, you are already half way done with your soap making process. To help you, there is a saponification chart with previously mentioned oils. Good luck!

Lipid	**Saponification**	Sodium hydroxide (NAOH)	Potassium hydroxide

			(KOH)
Avocado Oil	177 - 198	**0.134**	**0.188**
Avocado Oil	177 - 198	**0.134**	**0.188**
Apricot Kernel Oil	180 - 200	**0.135**	**0.19**
Almond Oil, Sweet	190 - 200	**0.139**	**0.195**
Aloe Vera Butter	220 - 260	**0.171**	**0.24**

Apricot Kernel Butter	130 - 145	**0.098**	**0.138**
Peanut Oil	**190**	**0.135**	**0.19**
Olive Oil	184 - 196	**0.135**	**0.19**
Cocoa Oil	173 - 188	**0.129**	**0.181**
Castor Oil	177 - 185	**0.129**	**0.181**
Jojoba, Natural	90 - 95	**0.066**	**0.093**

Chapter 7: Main Ingredients

Without lye, there is no soap.

One of the scariest aspects of soap making is working with lye. Lye – also popularly referred to as sodium hydroxide – is a compulsory part of producing your own handmade soap. In the absence of lye, there can never be a soap. Before a soap can be formed, fat must be present – your soap production butter and oil– and alkali, which in this case is sodium hydroxide must also be present before you can produce soap. When all these components are added together, they undergo a chemical reaction that is known as **saponification**. The lye is employed for the conversion of fats into soap; if this process is properly managed, there will never be a trace of lye in the resulting soap. Although it is possible to avoid the use of lye, all you need to do is to buy bases that are already pre-made. However, it is not advisable to follow this route as a result of the poor quality of soap produced when pre-made bases are used instead of lye. If you are hoping to make soap with a certain quality, the best means of achieving this is to draw up the exact type of soap you have in mind by using the right ingredient into the soap recipe.

Yes, lye can be a little dangerous if not properly handled. However, once you take your time to follow the laid down instructions in this book, lye is not as terrifying as you had earlier imagined. Different tutorials on soap production tend to be very cautious when dealing with lye; most of them portray lye as a frightening chemical. The truth here, of course, is that it is not dangerous or harmful so far you have a proper idea of the soap production process, and you follow simple safety guidelines — precautions as simple as what is obtainable in high school chemistry class.

So make sure you buy safety goggles, hand protection such as gloves, and you can add a fancy new apron just in case you decide to share some cute pictures with your friends on social media. The gloves and goggles and gloves can be bought at the local hardware store closest to your location, and there is also a higher probability that you will find the lye you need in the same store. It is important to note that many hardware stores have since increased the prices of lye to almost double what was obtainable just a few years ago AND it is almost impossible to see them on the shelf as most of these stores now keep their lye behind the counter. This is majorly due to a sudden surge in the abuse of methamphetamine, and lye is quite important when it comes to making meth. In actual facts, this can make it quite hard to source for lye, especially if the hardware in your locality decides to exclude it from their inventory.

Since hardware stores are no longer selling Red Devil Lye, one of the most common brands of lye that can found in most local stores is Roebic Heavy Duty Crystal Drain Opener. It is normally available in 2 lb. Containers and made up of 100% lye (caustic soda and sodium hydroxide). There are several other lye producers that are also excellent choices, and they will work fine so far they are at least 99% or purer. Another alternative means of getting high-quality lye is to reach out to other local soap producers and ask them where you can purchase lye locally with ease and/or if they have any spare lye you can buy to get started. Furthermore, recent advancements in technology now make it possible to buy lye over the internet from several companies that supply chemicals, soap production supplies, and Amazon. One of the advantages of buying from a chemical supplying company is that it gives you the chance to buy it in bulk. You can make the purchase according to your specification and needs, and your order can be picked up from these company's warehouse at an agreed date after payment has been finalized. Unless you are going to bulk production of soap, it is recommended to order just the amount of lye that is required for your soap making process.

Now that you know how to source for your lye, fully kitted with your safety goggles, gloves, and that fancy apron, you still need a few housewares. There is a higher probability that you already have a few of these things lying around in your home somewhere, so relax you not spending all your savings on this equipment. Because to be honest with you, the bulk of the money to be spent during a soap making process are expenses splurged on the purchase of the required ingredient. On second thought, if you feel like soap making is going to be an everyday thing, it is better to buy all new equipment in bids to keep the kitchen pots and utensils for food separate from the tools needed for the soap production process. While there is nothing wrong with using the same equipment for making soap and cooking spaghetti, just make sure the utensil is thoroughly washed to ensure there are no traces of the soap and you are good to go. You can also save some extra bucks by taking the time to check out stores that sell second-hand items. Without further ado, let us dive straight into the equipment you will need without a doubt:

A digital kitchen scale has the capability to take weight in ounces and grams that can also take care of more significant weight. I will recommend a Baker's Math scale, and these are usually durable as it tends to be accurate even after years of steady use and last much longer.

A stainless steel pot will be used for the mixing of the soap. Make sure you stay away from anything aluminium when it comes to hand made soap production.

This is because aluminium will undergo a chemical reaction with lye, and this is a chemical reaction that is not needed for soap production, and it can also be dangerous. Thus if you are not 100 per cent certain that the pot is not made with aluminium, it is recommended that you buy a new one that is made of steel.

A thermometer, like a candy thermometer, this will give you the chance to accurately determine the temperature of the lye-water and oils before mixing them together.

A hand blender or stick blender or immersion blender is required. It is known by different names, but basically, they are serving the same purpose. This executes the hardest physical part of soap production – the mixing. Due to this, the soap will trace faster, reducing the amount of time you have to spend mixing, and it also aids in ensuring that the batch of soap is evenly mixed.

Measuring cups and pitchers. It is imperative to have a large Pyrex measuring cup or a pitcher measuring cup to weigh out ingredients as well as to mix the lye-water in. Some soap producers do not make use of Pyrex glass measuring cups to mix the lye-water as it can etch the glass with time which will lead to the eventual breakage of the glass. However, it is possible to experience the same phenomenon with plastic pitchers after a long period of use. So, the decision of going for a glass pitcher or a plastic pitcher is entirely in your court. However, regardless of the container, you decide to use, ensure you inspect the containers periodically for any signs of wear or tear, in the case of a container breakage during the soap making process, ensure you mix the lye-water in a sink or outside.

It is also vital to have utensils such as a spatula or a big mixing spoon within reach. Make use of a long plastic spoon — to mix my lye water. A heavy-duty metal spoon to bring out jars of butter or oils that are semi-solid, and a spatula to scoop out all the soap from the pot into the mould.

You can make use of a grater or a knife to cut hard oils or butter into the required size.

You will discover what tools best suit your style with over, and it is quite possible that you already have these tools in your store or kitchen just lying fallow.

What about soap moulds?

Finally, it is vital to get a mould for the soap. You do not have to spend a huge sum of cash on a fancy soap producing mould. A soap mould can be made from everyday materials such as a Tupperware container lined with a trash bag or a cardboard box. Alternately, you can go for a silicone loaf pan (it is also used for baking) or you visit the local hardware store and get materials to make a wooden loaf soap mould. Using a wooden loaf soap mould is recommended because they are practically indestructible as such they last longer than other types of moulds. Most of the homemade soap recipes you are likely to create will fit perfectly inside these moulds. Do not forget that there is some preparation that is needed before making use of a wooden soap mould. While the silicone mould makes it possible to pour your soap into it directly, a wooden soap mould must be properly lined (this is also applicable when using a cardboard box or a Tupperware container). Empty cans of Pringles can be used as moulds for soaps that are round, simply remove the paper container from the soap after undergoing the saponification process. When the wooden soap mould is not lined, the soap will get stuck becoming quite hard to remove, and this can lead to unnecessary frustration.

You can cut and use parchment paper when lining the moulds. Just like wrapping a present, the paper is folded in a similar manner, but the top remains open. You can also use contact paper as the lining of a wooden mould. However, the price of both the contact paper and parchment paper can be quite high in the long run. Also, making use of parchment or contact paper to line soap moulds can be energy-sapping and time-consuming. As a result of this, it is recommended that you use commercial office trash bags as lining for your wooden soap moulds. These are relatively affordable in most grocery stores. If you are more of a practical individual and not a perfectionist – and you do not care if there are little creases on the bottom or sides of the soap, then this method of lining up a wooden mould is for you. Additionally, if you have unmolded the soap, you can still use the trash bag for what it was created for in the first instance – trash. In bids to use a trash bag as a wooden soap mould, simply unfold the bag but make sure you do not open it. Place it in the mode and tape the edges of the mould where the trash bag folds over the mould with masking tape. Of course, the method you use to line your wooden mould is entirely your choice, and I will advise that you go with the lining method you are more comfortable with. Once the soap is set, you only need to bring out the soap from the mould and remove the liner, cut into small bars and give it time to cure.

Learning about soapmaking ingredients.

I am assuming that by now, you have all the equipment needed for soap production. It is time to place more emphasis on the ingredients for a soap recipe. When trying to make a soap via cold process soap, it is highly advisable to use a tested and real soap recipe instead of coming up with your own recipe. It is quite better if you understand some of the basic chemical reactions about the ingredient used, it will broaden your knowledge when you are to create a soap recipe later in the future. The fats or soap production jars of butter or oils play an important role in determining the properties a soap will have. For instance, three of the most widely used soap production oils, especially for the first-timers include – palm oil, coconut oil, and olive oil. Palm oil will produce a soap with a hard bar, but a stable lather, olive oil aids in the production of a moisturizing bar with a stable lather and coconut oil helps in the making of a hard, cleansing bar that produces a fluffy lather. Every one of these oils has its own unique saponification value which aids in determining the amount of lye to be utilized in the soap recipe before saponification can happen in a way that will lead to the production of soap. If the lye is too much, the soap produced will be an unusable soap bar. Not enough lye and the soap produced will be a really soft soap bar filled with excess oil.

How to create your own homemade soap recipes.

When drawing up your own handmade soap recipes, there are also several additional resources that are actually free to guide you through the process. For instance, lye calculation will come in very handy when trying to figure out the amount of lye needed in a soap making process based on the amount and kind of oils that will be used in the recipe. A simple google search can help you find several links to different lye calculators.

Oils You Can Use to Make Homemade Soap

Picking the best oils for your soap production process is usually the most important part when it comes to the creation of a perfect soap bar. Oils can be several forms (unsaturated, saturated, scenting fats and/or oil and super-fatting) and with each having a unique smell. It is vital that you have a proper understanding of their properties, especially if you are the type that likes to try new things and may want to experiment with different oils for different soap making process. Here are just a few of the most widely used oils for a soap making process:

Almond Oil (Sweet)

This is a light moisturizing oil that absorbs well, and it is useful when producing a soap with low lather, and it is efficient in soap production – put an ounce per pound of fats to the soap mix at trace (this is the word used at the stage where the lye/soap mixture starts to thickens).

Avocado Oil

Employed mainly for super-fatting (if oil or any other substance is added at this stage, the ingredient maintains its natural form and will not mix or blend with the mixture), avocado oil is a brilliant moisturizer, and its healing properties come to the fore when it is included in your batch. It is rich in vitamins E, A, and D, and it can be used as a base oil up to 30 %. Avocado oil is the go-to oil when producing baby soap, as this is usually in gentle soaps for an individual with sensitive skin.

Coconut Oil

This oil does all the magic for your soap as it leads to the production of a bubbly lather when the soap is finally ready for use. Make sure you do not use too much of this oil though because an excess of coconut oil will lead to the drying of the skin. It is used for the production of a white, very hard soap bar that lathers even when if you use hard water or seawater. Use between only 20 to 30% of coconut oil in your base oils.

Cottonseed Oil

While this aid in the production of a thick, generous, and long-lasting lather, it is advisable to use this sparingly as it gets spoiled quite easily, depending on the climatic condition. If you decide to go with this oil during a soap making process, it is recommended that you use it as a maximum of 25% of total base oils.

Evening Primrose Oil

It is quickly absorbed, and it provides the skin with essential fatty acids that are required to halt the growth of bacteria in its tracks and promote the presence of antibodies, this will give the skin a chance of fighting off inflammation or infection. Do not use it as an additive in soap bars that are produced for especially for oily skin. It is advisable to use 2 tablespoons per 5 pounds of soap, to be included at the trace stage.

Grapeseed Oil

This is a type of lightweight, moisturizing oil that can be absorbed easily by the skin, and this one does not have any greasy after-feel. It has a short shelf life as such it is advisable you treat it with rosemary oleoresin extract. Apply an ounce per pound at the trace stage.

Hazelnut Oil

A brilliant moisturizer for both lotions and soaps, but this oil has a shelf life of 3 to 4 months. It is recommended that you do not use more than 5% of this oil in your recipe, and it is advisable that rosemary oleoresin extract is added to the batch as this helps in the prevention rancidity in the soap.

Honey

Honey is clearly not an oil, but it can be included in the mix to aid in the retention of skin moisture – glycerin also works in a similar way. It is recommended that you add 2 tablespoons per pound of oil when the mixture hits the trace stage.

Jojoba

Basically used as a super-fatting oil, it is very efficient when it comes to moisturizing and conditioning the skin. It has numerous health benefits, especially for individuals will varying skin conditions like acne, spots, and psoriasis, it is recommended for oily and sensitive skin, but it is actually suitable for every skin type. Add one or two ounces per pound at the trace stage.

Lard

Mainly used as a base oil, lard is usually soft, and may not be the best when added to cold water. This should be added to vegetable oils, and it is advisable at 70% the maximum of total oils.

Patience, time and years of experience will give you the right knowledge regarding the right oil to use.

Chapter 8: The Nitty-Gritties Of Herbal Soap Making

Now that you know the difference between buying commercially produced, chemical laden soaps in the market and herbal soaps; as well as the benefits of making the herbal soaps yourself; it is time to get cooking. You must remember, however, that although accurate measurements are necessary, herbal soap making, is more of an art than a science. This means you do need to precise measurements but you can also have loads of fun. Let's start.

Herbal Soap Making Equipment

If you want to make your own herbal soaps at home, you will be pleased to find out that most of the tools and equipment are most probably in your kitchen already. And if they are not, they can easily be found and purchased online or in your local supermarket. In addition, basic soap making equipment do not cost a fortune.

To get started in making your own herbal soap, you will need the following supplies. It is highly recommended that you do not start making your herbal soap until you have all these tools handy so that you will not have any interruptions in the soap making process.

Safety equipment - Rubber gloves and safety goggles are imperative. These protect your hands and your eyes from the lye solution and the corrosive raw soap. You MUST have good safety equipment; so it is best to invest in high quality googles and gloves. Your hands and eyes will thank you for it.

An accurate scale - For any aspiring or professional soap maker, a high quality, accurate soap scale is an extremely important tool. Your scale should be able to measure in grams and ounces. The scale will be used to measure everything - the additives, fragrance, lye, oils, and even water. Without an accurate measurement, soap making will be unsuccessful.

Large Pyrex pitcher – If you would be making small batches (i.e. 2 to 3 lbs. of soap), start with a large Pyrex pitcher or a glass measuring cup with cover to mix everything in.

Stainless steel pot – If you will be making bigger batches, get an 8 to 12 quart stainless steel pot with a lid. This will serve as your mixing pot as well as your actual "Soap Pot", where the soap making will happen.

Pitcher – The pitcher will be used to mix up the lye solution. For herbal soap making, get yourself a 2 to 3 quart, heat-resistant stainless steel pitcher with a lid. Make sure you clearly label it (i.e. "Danger Lye. Do not touch.").

Another pitcher —You need another 2 to 3 quart heat-resistant glass bowl or pitcher to measure and hold the liquid oils before adding them to the soap pot.

Stirring spoon - A big stainless steel spoon is necessary for stirring the lye solution.

Thermometer - A precise, quick reading thermometer is required to monitor the temperature of the melted oils and the lye solution.

Measuring spoons - Stainless steel measuring spoons for measuring fragrance or essential oils, colorants and/or other ingredients.

Several small beakers, bowls, or measuring cups – This would be used to hold the essential oils, herbs, colorants, separated soap, and other ingredients.

Spoons or small whisks – These will be used to mix the fragrance oils and colorants with the melted oil before adding them to the Soap Pot.

Large stainless steel ladle – This will be used to ladle out the mixture and for stirring, too.

Blender – You could use either a hand-held immersion or stick blender to mix the oils with the lye and start the saponification process.

Soap Mold – You can opt for basic molds or go crazy with different shapes and sizes. You can choose from commercial soap molds, yogurt cups, shoe boxes or any container that is leak-proof and made of glass or stainless steel. You can also use cardboard or wood molds as long as you line it with heavy duty freezer paper first.

Rubber spatulas – For scraping any remaining bits of soap from the pot.

Paper towels or dishcloths – For wiping spills.

This is a good starting set that would accommodate basic herbal soap projects. As you make more batches, you will be able to tailor your equipment to fit your specific soap making style.

Important Reminders

Avoid using anything made of aluminum, iron, tin, or Teflon because lye will corrode them.

Avoid using plastic because the heat will melt them.

Lye also corrodes wood tools and utensils over time.

Before you Begin

Do not multitask. Disruptions during the process of making soap lead to accidents.

Safety first. Lye is extremely caustic and can burn your eyes, skin and equipment upon contact. Make sure you have protective clothing, and heavy duty googles and gloves. Protective gear is MANDATORY.

Prepare all the equipment and ingredients before you begin.

Do not rush. Accuracy matters. Take your time in measuring the ingredients before you begin. Measure the ingredients by weight ounces and not fluid ounces.

Handle lye and certain essential oils with care. Make sure you have running water and vinegar handy, in case of lye spills. Vinegar neutralizes lye.

If a spill does happen, attend to your skin first. Rinse the affected area with cool water for more than 5 continuous minutes. Apply vinegar and rinse again. If the burn is severe, go to the emergency room ASAP.

Store all soap making substances and equipment in a safe place that is inaccessible to children.

Label all soap making substances and equipment properly. Do not use them for anything else.

A well-ventilated work area is a must because mixtures of lye and oils will produce fumes.

A heat proof work table is also a must because when lye is added to water; the mixture will reach 150 to 200°F.

Educate your family about soap making and its hazards. Instruct them not to go anywhere near your equipment and supplies.

Rule of thumb. Always the lye crystals to cold water and never the other way around. Adding water to lye crystals could result to an explosion. Common sense is key. Practice Safety. First procedures and CLAY Go (Clean as you go.) Never leave the work area unattended.

Chapter 9: Basic Techniques In Making Your Soap Bar Or Liquid Soap

Okay, you currently have the entirety of your gear and fixings. It is currently an ideal opportunity to choose which cycle of soap making you might want to utilize. In this part, you will figure out how each cycle functions and the advantages and downsides of each. To start with, there are two or three things you should know for all methods.

Significantly, you start by finding an all-around ventilated zone to work in. When you discover, that spread your workspace. You can utilize towels, a paper, or expendable decorative liner. The reason for this is to secure the region and take into consideration sheltered, simple cleanup. At that point, you have to put on elastic gloves and security goggles on the off chance that you will be making a soap that utilizes lye. You should likewise have the entirety of your materials prepared first. The entirety of the fixings ought to be actually estimated and in their suitable compartments before beginning to make the soap. Ensure all the fixings and hardware you will require in later stages is good to go. If fundamental, line your molds. It is likewise fitting to peruse your formula completely before you start. Ensure you comprehend the strategies you will be performing and the fixings just as the hardware you will utilize.

The remainder of this section will disclose to you a progression of cycles that can be utilized to make soap. The virus cycle, hot cycle, liquefy and pour, and rebatching strategies will be shrouded inside and out. Directions for how to make fluid soap and whipped soap will likewise be given.

The Cold Process

The principal usually utilized method of making soap is utilizing the virus cycle. The upside of the virus cycle is that there is a short 'dynamic' creation time (around 60 minutes). The soap made is commonly smoother and even in surface than that created utilizing different methods. Because of the way that less lye is utilized in this cycle contrasted and the hot cycles, this kind of soap will in general be gentler on the skin. The burden is that cool prepared soaps need to a solution for four to about a month and a half before utilizing so the compound change can finish.

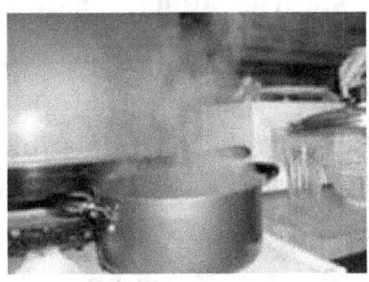

The initial step is to make a water and lye blend. While picking your formula, it will determine how much lye and how much water to consolidate. A decent dependable guideline if your formula doesn't show a particular sum is to utilize 1-section lye, 3-section water proportion. It is critical to quantify the lye by weight and ideally measure it into a compartment that you can shut if you have to delay or your work interferes.

Significant wellbeing note: When consolidating add the lye to the water and not water to the lye for security purposes. If the water is added to lye, there will be a substance response much like putting vinegar and preparing soft drinks together. A holder that can withstand high temperatures must be utilized for blending because the synthetic response between the lye and the water will make the blended warmth to around 200 degrees.

When the lye has been added to the water, mix persistently until the lye is broken up or the required response won't happen when you blend this mix in with the oil or fat. When joined, place a thermometer in the holder and put it in a safe spot.

The subsequent advance is to set up your corrosive. On the off chance that you are utilizing a strong fat, dissolve it to the fluid-structure. Measure your fats or oils into your soap skillet utilizing a scale. Combine the fixings, placed a thermometer in, and put in a safe spot.

Right now is an ideal opportunity to get both of your blends to a temperature of around 95 degrees. This is most effortlessly done by placing the lye compartment into cold water or an ice shower. You may likewise decide to warm your fat over the oven or in the microwave at little augmentations. At the point when they are both the necessary comparable temperature, empty the lye blend into the fat gradually while mixing. It is significant that you don't quit blending until you come to the 'follow' stage. On the off chance that you choose to hand blend, you ought to accomplish follow in around 45 minutes. On the off chance that you utilize a stick blender, you can arrive at following in as meager as 2 minutes. When utilizing a stick blender you would prefer not to turn it on and let it get down to business. Rather, exchange beats with blending movements while the blender is off. You realize you have the correct consistency or have arrived at the following when you can utilize your spoon to sprinkle a portion of the substance on the head of the rest and it remains there for a piece before sinking. Remember that the time it takes to accomplish follow can change broadly relying upon temperature, mixing technique, and sorts of fats utilized.

When the following stage has arrived at then aroma, shading, and whatever else you needed to include can be blended in. Consolidate added substances totally and fill molds. Spread the molds with a cover and enclose them by 6-8 towels. No warmth should escape as it is required for the saponification cycle to finish. Leave them to fix and cool for 18-36 hours.

Next, eliminate the soap from the molds. This is an ideal opportunity to slice if you have chosen to make bar soaps. Spot the soaps on a cooling rack. Flip them each 6-8 days. The soap ought to be completely restored in 4 a month and a half. Encompassing the soap with outdoors and permitting it to solidify and age as the synthetic responses stop finishes this relieving cycle.

The Hot Process

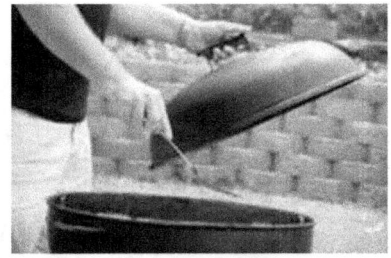

Hot cycle soap is more suggestive of prior occasions and of how soap would probably have been initially made. There are a few points of interest and disservices to this procedure. The main bit of leeway is that you include scent and shading after the saponification cycle has happened hence changing their properties practically nothing. The hot handled soap is frequently somewhat milder making it simpler to cut. Then again, the hot prepared soap isn't too simple to form, and getting a smooth top layer is troublesome. Additionally, the way toward cooking utilizes power and vitality assets not needed by the virus cycle. It is conceivable to utilize an oven, twofold heater, or Crockpot to make hot handled soap.

Likewise, with the virus cycle, you need to make your lye and water blend in one holder and your liquidized oils and fats in another pot. You don't need to hold up until they arrive at a specific temperature to join them when utilizing this strategy. What you need to see when combining them is partition. You plan to see yellowish curds on the last, a thick layer of oil in the center, and white froth on the top. When you see these layers, put the pot over low warmth and mix ceaselessly (either by hand or with blender). If you don't mix, the arrangement will bubble over onto the oven or counter. This is risky and one reason you are wearing a wellbeing outfit and have materials to tidy up lye close by. Cook the soap until you get bubbles that are about the size of the top of a pi. This should take around 15-25 minutes. Eliminate the soap from the warmth and let it cool until you don't perceive any air pockets, around 10 minutes. Warm on low until bubbles return. Cool again till bubbles are no more. Rehash this until no layers are left and the blend you have is even and uniform. It ought to help you to remember Vaseline. Include scent, shading and some other wanted added substances. Immerse your molds. There is no compelling reason to protect your molds as the saponification cycle has just happened. When the soap is cool you can eliminate it from molds. If necessary this is the ideal opportunity to cut the soap. Hot prepared soap can solution however long you feel essential. There is inconsistency among soap producers regarding whether hot cycle soap should be restored at all while some reserve relieving for 4 a month and a half. It is fitting to permit probably some relieving time with the soap on cooling racks.

Melt and Pour

The softened and pour strategy is exceptionally well known with apprentices. Utilizing this procedure isn't really soap appearing well and good because there is no saponification cycle. Rather, glycerin is joined with surfactants to make a soap base that can be industrially bought. Even though this cycle doesn't need the logical ability that different cycles do, it permits the soap producer to focus on the style of the soap and the outcome can smell incredible and be genuinely wonderful. One of the significant advantages of this method is having the option to evade the utilization or cruel synthetics, for example, lye. This is especially covetous to soap creators with kids or pets who oftentimes enter the soap making zone. Utilizing this strategy is an extraordinary method to get youngsters engaged with soap making. To make liquefy and pour soap, start by softening your bought soap base. This should be possible in a microwave, Crockpot, or twofold kettle. At that point, include any added substances, hues, or aromas you wish. Presently empty the soap into your form and let it solidify. When it's hard, remove it from the shape and let it dry on cooling racks for a few days before utilizing it.

Rebatching

Rebatching, additionally called the hand-processed strategy, is the last cycle of making strong soaps that we will discuss. The advantages of this cycle are setting aside cash and lessening waste from not really lovely clumps of soap. It is likewise an approach to resuscitate old soap that has lost its aroma. Since no crude synthetic concoctions are included, kids can help make this sort of soap.

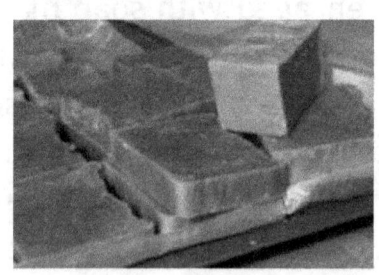

The initial phase in this procedure includes making a plain soap utilizing either the hot or cold cycle. Use soap to which no botanicals, colors, or scents have been included. After the soap is solidified, grind it with a blade or cheddar grater held for the reason. Spot the ground soap in a little warmth verification holder to microwave or put it into a scaled-down Crockpot or a twofold heater. Include nine ounces of water for every twelve ounces of soap and dissolve it tenderly and slowly. It is significant when utilizing this procedure to work with little groups inside little holders so the soap doesn't consume. Try not to permit the blend to bubble and be mindful so as not to mix an excessive amount of because bubbles and air pockets are probably going to create. When the soap is liquefied, let it cool to around 150 degrees. Now include your botanicals, scents, hues, and so on. Now it is ready to be poured into molds. Once it is cooled, remove it from the molds. Slice if necessary and place on cooling racks for several days before storing.

Liquid Soap

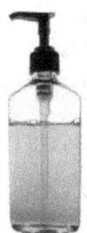

A few people like to have fluid soap for washing hands as opposed to a strong bar. Fluid soap likewise has the advantage of being prepared to use in around 3 days rather than 3 weeks.

The main method to make fluid soap is to follow the formula for a basic soap made with the virus cycle. Adhere to the guidelines as per the formula you need to utilize. Ensure it gets well past a follow before embellishment. Rather than restoring your soap as guided, it will just sit for around three days at that point follow these means:

Remove the soap from the shape

Shave, slash, or mesh it. Ensure you use gloves for this cycle as the soap is as yet harsh.

Mix 1 cup of the soap pieces with the picked scents, colors, and so on.

Put the blend in a twofold evaporator or slow cooker with 3 cups of water.

Melt the soap steadily while mixing.

Break up any bunches with a plastic whisk or fork. You may locate that a few pieces don't dissolve. If so you should strain the blend later.

Once the soap has dissolved to a point you believe is suitable, scoop some out and permit it to cool in a water shower. It ought to be runny when cooled.

If it is excessively thick, you can include more water.

If it isn't sufficiently thick, you can include additional soap pieces.

10. Reheat varying to get the correct surface.

11. Once you feel it's prepared, strain the soap into a holder.

The other strategy for making fluid soap includes a broiler. The cycle is like creation a hot cycle bar soap aside from it utilizes an alternate sort of lye. Rather than utilizing sodium hydroxide, the fluid soap utilizes potassium hydroxide. To cause hot cycle fluid soap, to follow this system:

Mix your lye-water arrangement and set it to cool (notice potassium hydroxide will get more smoking more immediately when blended in with water than sodium hydroxide).

Mix your fats and oils.

Blend the lye arrangement with the oils in a broiler-safe pot until it arrives at follow. This could take for some time with fluid soap yet you will see that when follow begins, the soap thickens rapidly

Cover the pot with a spread that fits safely.

Put the pot in a 180-degree broiler.

Cook for 4-5 hours blending every 20-30 minutes.

When the soap is genuinely clear, eliminate it from the broiler.

The glue now should be weakened. Bring 40 oz. of refined water to a bubble.

Add the water to the soap.

10. Stir it in.

11. Put the cover on the pot and hold up about 60 minutes.

12. Stir.

13. Put the cover on for the time being and mix again in the first part of the day.

14. Add aroma and shading.

15. Let rest.

16. Store and appreciate.

Whipped Soap

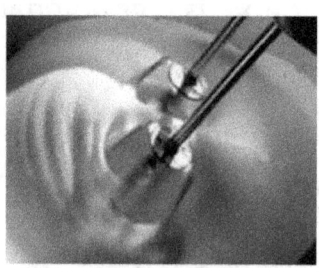

The whipped soap is a pleasant minor departure from the virus cycle of soap making. The outcome is eccentric soap looking like meringues, mists, and puffs of whipped cream. To make whipped soap follow these means:

Find a formula with a level of hard oils (a.k.a. coconut, palm, grease, fat, palm portion, shea margarine, cocoa spread, shortening) that is more prominent than 80%.

Weigh out your hard oils and spot in a glass blending bowl.

Whip the entirety of the oils with a hand blender until tops structure.

Slowly include the fluid oils.

Whip for a few minutes to accomplish tops once more.

Add the lye-water arrangement your formula calls for to the oils several tablespoons one after another.

Keep whipping

And whip some more

Add aroma remembering that this will diminish your pinnacles a piece.

10. Depending on the oils utilized, the soap will be done when it takes after thick yogurt, delicate serve frozen yogurt, whipped spread, cream cheddar, or whipped egg whites.

11. Add shading.

12. Mold. Whipped soap works best in 'sliceable' molds. You can likewise utilize the soap to "ice" or line plans onto other arranged soaps as you would a cake or treat.

13. Whipped soap will take at any rate 24 if not 36 hours to set.

14. Let its solution for a little while.

Cleaning up

Since your soap is made, the time has come to tidy up. Ideally, you worked in a sorted out manner and no spills were making the cleanup cycle a lot simpler. When cleaning, recollect that lye is presently in a few spots, 2 pots, and any devices that you utilized for blending. It could likewise be on your gloves, the thermometer, and the scale. It is as yet risky and scathing because it didn't need to chance to respond with fat and saponify. The crude soap is harsh so be cautious while tidying up. The initial step is to manage the extra crude soap. Utilize an elastic spatula to scratch the soap out of your pot and into your molds, the less clean you have in your pot the simpler it will be to clean. Presently flush the entirety of your compartments and apparatuses. Wipe your pot out with paper towels and discard them right away. It is additionally conceivable to utilize "shop" towels, simply forget about them short-term before placing them in the clothes washer so the saponification cycle from the extra fixings will finish and no substance responses will happen in the clothes washer. Then again, you can utilize a great deal of high temp water and "genuine" soap to wash the pot. You could likewise put the entirety of your devices requiring cleaning into the pot, spread it with a top, and leave it overnight. By the following morning, the oils and lye that had remained will be a soap. Simply tidy it up in the sink and dry. Try not to wash your materials in your dishwasher; the response will make water pour out onto your floor.

Storing soap

After your soap has restored, a proper method to store it must be found. Remember that the time span of the usability of handcrafted soap is substantially less than economically made soap and turns out to be significantly shorter on the off chance that it isn't put away appropriately. Custom made soap can last about a year when kept in a cool, dry spot. Setting it in an impenetrable holder that is put in a dim, dry, cool spot is ideal. When you start to utilize your soap, it is critical to keep it as dry as conceivable so it endures longer.

Chapter 10: A Little More Insight Into The Ingredients

Before we move on to showcasing some amazing recipes for making soap, we must also go over some of the most common ingredients in the making of the soap process, what their purpose is, and how they can be altered to suit your soap wishes.

Sodium Hydroxide or Lye

Lye is the most crucial element of the entire soap making process. You simply cannot make any soap without it. Because soap is made with the help of a chemical process, which is part of the base of everything that you are going to make with your soap recipes and ideas. You have to use Sodium Hydroxide in order to make soap, however, if you are not yet ready to use this chemical, you can purchase the pre-made soap base and just melt it in a pot.

Water

Water is important in the initial stages of the soap making process where all the ingredients are mixed together. The water is what helps all of the ingredients come together and form into a pleasant, smooth mixture. However, the water will eventually evaporate, whether you warm up the soap mixture or you leave it for a few weeks to dry on its own. When you use water, you need to expect that your soap will eventually shrink from the original size of the mold that you used when you were shaping your soap. Make sure that you always use the correct amount of water that is shown in the recipe, you must make sure that your water amounts are correct so that you have the mixture that you expect to have for your soap.

Fats and Oils

Essentially, any oil or fat can be used to make soap. You can be as diverse as you want to be in this sense, because all oils will eventually harden into the proper soap mixture as long as you make sure that all of the ingredients are at their correct proportions. However, it is very unlikely that only one type of oil or fat will be used for a single soap. This is because using only one type of soap or fat would make the soap very one-dimensional and it would also reduce the effectiveness of the soap and the healthy benefits that would come from it.

You can sometimes also play around with the oils or fats by adding an extra layer to the soap at the end of the process. This extra layer will not mix with the rest of the ingredients, which will make the soap get more moisturizing qualities and help to take care of your skin better. However, if you are only just starting out, don't worry too much about the oil or the fat, and instead stick to the precise recipe until you feel more confident in creating your own.

The most common oils to use when making your own soap

Oils are going to be one of the most exciting things about making your own soap. You can mix and match them to get amazing scents and also many different health properties for your skin. There are practically no limits when it comes to mixing the oils together, and the more experience you gather making soap, the better you will be about being original in your own soap making.

The following are some of the most popular oils that are used when making soap. Try and learn about them as much as possible, because the chemistry of the oils will help you to decide what you want your soap to include and how you want it to help the people who will be using it.

Beeswax

This is one of the most popular ingredients for people who have sensitive, dry skin that needs a lot of help to be moisturized again. You probably already know that beeswax is one of the most popular ingredients in lip products, which is why you should definitely consider it in your own soap recipes. But this ingredient won't just make your soap great for the skin, it will also help to make the soap much harder than other oils would, which means that the soap bar will last for a longer period of time. It also helps to keep large batches of soap firm and easy to cut into pieces.

Cocoa Butter

This is another butter that is great for moisturizing skin. It also has a delicious smell and is very popular for soap bars that are made for bedtime and for the colder seasons. However, make sure that you do not use a lot of cocoa butter in your own recipes. Although it will help to harden the soap, it will also melt very quickly when it comes in contact with water when used, so if there is too much of this ingredient in your soap then it will make the soap bar crumble and fall apart. Instead, use it in smaller quantities to add a touch of healthy moisture and scent to your soap bar.

Coconut Oil

This is a great oil to add to any kind of soap bar. Coconut oil is super healthy for your skin, and it is also a great oil to use for soap bars that are intended to wash hair, because coconut oil will also hydrate hair follicles better than any other oil that is currently available. Also, coconut oil added to soap will produce a lovely foam when used, which will help to really get the feeling of using a soap bar when washing. It is completely organic, and it can even be used for soap bars that are intended for pets (although make sure that you follow the recipe very carefully).

Olive Oil

For centuries, olive oil has been the heart and soul of the Mediterranean. It is no wonder that it is so popular, because its healing properties are enormous and can be applied to any part of the human body. This is a great oil to use for very sensitive skin that needs to be deeper conditioned. This oil has a very distinct smell, so it is best not to use it in recipes that need to have a particular scent because the olive oil is likely to overpower them.

Palm Oil

This is a very popular soap ingredient, however, it is one that has become very controversial over the years, so if you are going to use it, you need to make sure that you keep nature at the back of your mind. The problem with palm oil is the way that it is produced. Many forests have been destroyed and many animals left without their home (especially orangutans) because of the way that this oil is produced. This is why many people are stepping away from the use of palm oil in their soap making process. However, there are still palm oils that are very careful about the environment and that are marked with the 'sustainable' label. This means that the production of this particular palm oil has not cause any harm to nature or animals in the process.

Soybean Oil

This oil doesn't have that many healthy ingredients for skin, but it does provide a lot of conditioning. It is best used in combination with other oils, because it will add another element of conditioning without any kind of scent. So, if you want to include deep moisturizing without ruining the original scent that you were planning on adding to your soap bar, then soybean oil is a great one to use.

Shea Butter

This is another fat that is very popular in skincare products. And it is no wonder that this is the case because shea butter has an amazing smell as well as great moisturizing properties. However, this is one fat that is actually very difficult to turn into soap. This is because it breaks down very easily, which means that no matter what shape you wanted your soap to have, shea butter will probably ruin it. However, when you become more experienced in soap making, you can add measured quantities of this fat to your soap for an extra layer of smell and moisture without actually ruining the structure of your soap.

Sweet Almond Oil

This is similar to shea butter because it will also cause the structure of your soap to fall apart. Sweet almond oil is great for some added moisture and it also feels very light in the soap. However, it should only be added as a special ingredient in small quantities. Also, almond oil has its own scent, so be careful when you decide to mix it with other scents because it might cause a confusion.

Great antioxidants to add to your soap

Antioxidants are not added to soap recipes to provide you with extra healthy elements. In fact, they are added to recipes in order to make the entire soap mixture more stable, and to create a more beautiful-looking soap bar. Normally, when you work with wet products (which is what the original soap mixture is) you would expect to use preservatives in order to protect the quality of the product. However, this is not the case with soap because the water that you use for it (which is the home of potential bacteria) will entirely evaporate by the time that the soap bar is ready to use.

This is where antioxidants come in to help you along the way. Their job is to make sure that the free-floating oils inside your soap are stable and that they don't become rancid over time. Soap bars do have a long period of use; however, you don't want to keep them for years because the ingredients will start to turn bad.

Antioxidants are used as the very last step of the process of making soap. A small quantity of an antioxidant is added to the mixture at the very end and must be measured carefully so that it doesn't disturb the wanted texture of the soap. There are basically two main antioxidants that any soap maker will use.

(GSE) Grapefruit seed extract

This is a great antioxidant to ensure that the oils inside your soap mixture do not spoil for a very long time. It is also very popular because it will not add any additional scent to the mixture, and the quantities are very easy for beginners to measure.

(ROE) Rosemary Oleoresin Extract

This is also a great antioxidant to use, however, it is usually one that is used by professionals. Its texture is very thick, which means that it is more difficult to measure the correct amount that is needed for one particular recipe. Also, it has a very strong rosemary scent. Although rosemary can be mixed with other scents to make interesting scent combinations, you should not use this antioxidant in your recipe if you don't want any rosemary scent in your soap.

Chapter 11: Soap Making Process

Now to the moment we have been waiting for; how to make that sweet-scented soap!

There are two processes; hot and cold.

Cold process:

This process is the most common methods used to make soap. Soaps are made using oil and lye. The correct amount of fats/oils and lye are what make a great soap when using cold process. Use the saponification chart provided in this book, or you can look up on others to show you which ratios to use. This is to help you not have too much hydroxide in your soap or excess fat.

To work this out properly;

- the oil specification value of each unique fat is checked first on the saponification chart, which shows the precise saponification value of the fat.

- The value should then be converted into the equivalent of sodium hydroxide value. This is critical for extra lye creates a high pH that can irritate the skin.

- The lye is mixed in water and oils heated if they are at room temperature.

- The two are mixed afterward to the point of emulsification. This is the thickening of the mixture or known as a trace. It is affected by the type of additives you have used. Light trace forms when you use herbs, oatmeal or other solid additives but heavy trace occurs after adding essential and fragrance oils.

- This is then poured into molds and kept warm using towels and left for 24 to 48 hours. Milk soaps and other soaps that have sugar do not need insulation as the presence of sugar speeds up producing heat.

- If you notice your soap turns translucent then dark again, it is okay. The soap is going through a gel phase.

- After insulation process, the soap is unmolded and cut into shapes and ready for use.

Let the cold process soap cure and harden for 2 to 6 weeks after cutting into bars to make the lye saponify and excess water evaporates.

To speed up your soap making process, less water or better known as a discount is used.

For most people, this process results in a smoother soap that the hot process.

Hot process:

This process has been there since the first soap was made by the Babylonians. You use heat from either a crock pot or a double boiler, like the olden days where soap is cooked for a period of time till the process of saponification is complete.

This method is ideal for a busy person who does not want to wait several weeks for the soap to be ready for use. The heat allows the soap to be used immediately it is made.

A discount is not required when using this process due to the amount of water that is used in the extra cooking time. The consistency is not like that of the cold process as the soap is lumpy and after making it, the soap is soft.

In this process:

- Hydroxide and fat are both heated at approximately $80\text{-}100^\circ$ C until the completion of the saponification process. As a beginner, you need to research how to notice if saponification has taken place.

- The best part about this is not needing to know the amount of hydroxide to use. It is not limited to sodium hydroxide only but involves potash or wood ashes as well.

- When saponification is confirmed, the soap is precipitated from solution by adding salts to drain excess liquid. The liquid carries impurities from the fat and the color compounds then leave behind a pure batch of soap.

- The soap is then poured into molds and you can process the sodium hydroxide used to recover glycerin.

Cold Process Soaps

This process allows you to go all out in the creativity department as you control what ingredients you are going to use for your soap. You get to make weird looking soaps that have weird ingredients too, no judgment or regrets at all.

Extra oils and fats can be added in this process to your specifications, this is called "superfatting".

For beginners, it is advisable not to use this process until you have mastered the art of soap making. There are plenty of recipes that are superfatting or are already one.

For your first experiment with soap making, here are several recipes you can use:

1. 4.5lbs Soap recipe

16 ounces of Palm oil

16 ounces of Canola oil

16 ounces of Coconut oil

15.8 ounces of water

6.9 ounces of Lye (which is 5% super fatted)

Note: make sure you are wearing eye safety glasses, breathing mask and rubber gloves.

Instructions

Add lye to water and stir well till they have mixed properly. Beware that fumes are likely to be produced when you do this.

Set the mixture aside and let it cool until it reaches 110 Fahrenheit. place it in a well-ventilated area, or if you can't find one, put the mixture outside.

Take all the oils; canola, palm and coconut oil and melt them.

Give them time to cool to 110 Fahrenheit. Should be -5 or +5 degrees Fahrenheit than the temperature of the lye solution.

Add the lye/water mixture to your melted oil mixture making sure not to spill any.

Stir as vigorously as you can; the stick blender comes in handy here. Stir till you notice trace occurring. It will look similar to thin custard.

Once trace has formed, it is time to pour into chosen molds the mixture.

In 4 to 5 days, you can take them out of their molds and set them aside for 5 to 6 weeks to allow curing to occur and saponification to complete.

Congratulations! You have made your first batch of soap, that I'm certain smells incredible. Next, we learn to make soap using the hot process.

Hot Process Soaps

Concerns aired about this process is removal of soap from molds. Using wooden molds is easier than plastic mold.

You might notice your soap at first is sticky, but that is all right, let it sit out in open air for a couple of days and it will solidify properly.

Since you can use a crock pot or microwave, I'll show you a couple of recipes using both.

Hot process recipe using crock pot

You will require:

3 tbsp. of Honey

3 tbsp. of oat flour

32 ounces of olive oil

12 ounces of water

4.50 ounces of Lye (5% superfatting)

and

3 ounces of castor oil

Instructions

1. To your crock pot, preheat it first before you add the oils you are using to it.

2. While doing this, mix lye and water and do it with great care.

3. When the solution has blended and dissolved properly, add it to the oils in the crock pot as slowly and gently as you can.

4. Use a stick blender to blend it quickly to achieve a thick trace.

5. Cover your crock pot when you complete blending the mix and turn the heat to high.

6. After every 10 to 15 minutes, check your concoction and stir it properly each time, and replace the lid afterward.

7. To check if the soap is ready for the knife test, the soap must have risen and turned in on itself making it resemble mashed potatoes.

This is simply putting a clean knife into the mixture. These are usually the results:

- If the knife looks waxy when pulled out, try the next test, which is tongue.

- If it is still the same, add one tsp of olive oil and stir it in properly. Then allow it to cook for another 2 minutes.

8. Once it has passed the knife test, add the 3 tbsp. of honey and stir it in the mixture cooking.

9. The change of color should be immediate to a dark color. When you hear the soap sizzling, turn off your crock pot.

10. Take your oatmeal and mix it with 3 to 4 tbsp. of cold water (or if you'd like instead, add goat milk in place of water) and make sure it is not lumpy. Then add it to the soap mixture and stir generously.

11. Now you can add the mixture into molds. Approximately 1 quart of soap should be produced from this.

12. After 24 hours, your soap will be ready for cutting.

And you have yourself some sweet oat-smelling soap!

Now we **make soap without using Lye**, yes it seems far-fetched but quite achievable, but not entirely used (I'll explain). The end product will be free of chemicals and all natural, mainly based on your taste and what you would like it to look like.

Hand-milled soap or melt-pour soap is soap made without adding caustic soda. This is the explanation; the process of mixing lye and water has already been done when you are making this type of soap.

Your requirements will be:

Molds

A natural soap base

Plants or herbs

Essential oils and

Liquid

Double boiler or crock pot

● The natural soap should be without added chemicals and fragrances. Use cream or white colored soap as they are the best to work with when hand-milling.

● Plants can be either dried or fresh plants, like dried lavender or fresh rose petals. If you have plant powder, this will work as a natural colorant. Turmeric will turn the soap orange; Spirulina makes it green or the Himalayan pink salts that create a pink hue.

● Depending on the amount of soap you are melting, a bread pan can suffice. Make sure before you use it to line it with parchment paper if you are not using silicone molds.

- To prevent the soap from burning when you are melting it, the liquid will come in handy here. It can vary from water to green tea to coconut milk.

- Add 100% natural essential oils as they work great when hand milling. You can mix such essential oils as follows:

- Dried lavender with Plumeria oil

- Turmeric powder with Thyme oil

Instructions

Grate two regular bars of soap or 8 ounces of soap using a food processor or cheese grater and place it in a double boiler.

On it, add an ounce or two of whatever liquid you are going to use.

Set the heat on low and stir frequently to avoid burning the soap mixture. This can be as short as 15 minutes to an hour. When the liquid is lumpy and translucent, remove it from the heat.

Add the remaining ingredients- essential oils and plant or herbs.

Stir this to the consistency you like. Then pour it into molds.

Put your mold in the freezer for an hour. Let it cool and remove it from the mold.

Cut into shapes and sizes that you like using a food scraper.

If you used a lot of liquid, let the soap dry for several days. As the period of drying all depends on the amount of liquid used.

To extend the life of your soap, dry it thoroughly after use.

And there we have it, easy to make melt-and-pour liquid soap.

Re-Batching Soap

It is, if not, the simplest form of making soap. This is mainly used when making liquid soap. All you require is

Leftover soap

Milk or water

Coconut milk or goat milk (as an option to add)

You will:

Take your leftover soap, about 4 ounces, cut them up into tiny pieces or you can grate them.

Heat about a gallon of distilled water until steam comes off.

Add to the hot water your grated or chopped soap.

Take the mixture off the heat and let it cool for 15 minutes.

Re-blend the mixture using a hand blender and allow it to sit overnight.

If you have some goat milk or coconut milk lying around, add some into this soap mixture and blend.

N.B: Make sure your mixture is properly blended, if not, continue blending till the consistency is right.

When done, put the soap in liquid hand containers and refill when necessary.

These are just a couple of recipes that show how hot and cold processes vary.

Making Transparent Soap

That colorful looking soap that is almost clear, an example is Lifebuoy. The soap smells great and for most people, especially kids, they love how they look.

Transparent soap is part solvent part soap. There are crystals that form in your soap when sodium hydroxide is used. The crystals are the reason behind the opaque color of the soap. To make it transparent it the fun part and pretty easy.

Dissolving your soap of choice in enough liquid to make the crystals small enough that you will be able to see through it, making it appear transparent.

The process is pretty long and will take quite a while to make the soap, approximately half a day. Therefore, make sure you the time to start and complete the process but anyway here is the process.

You will need:

An oven

A clear Pyrex cup

5 spoons

Spray bottle of ethanol

A whisk and a stick blender

Large pot, one with a spout or a crock pot o

Essential oil of choice or a fragrance oil

Saran wrap

Breathing mask

A plastic strainer and

Litmus paper for testing pH level

Instructions

Measure out the essential oils you have selected, mix and heat them while using a slow cooker. The cooker should be able to hold 5 liters.

Now to make the lye, use 170 grams of water and sodium hydroxide (NaOH). put it to the side to cool.

Measure the oil and lye temperature to make sure they are at about $60^{\circ}C$, then pour the lye into the oil mixture and stir. Use a stick blender.

Within a couple of minutes, you will notice trace on the soap mixture. At this point cover it with a tight lid. Pop your oven open and place it in with your oven heated at 80°C for an hour and a half.

There is the option of you leaving your soap mixture in the pot you used on warm, then after an hour and a half to make sure that the next stage is the gel stage. A few hours are all it needs to achieve this; do try to reduce your water loss as much as you can.

The soap will be fairly neutral at 1 $^1/_2$ hours to 2 hours. It should be in the gels stage at this moment. The pH at this level is between a nine and ten.

Use the litmus paper to check the pH level. Dissolve a tiny bit of the soap in a small amount of water and use the litmus paper to get the correct readings. The pH of your soap should be neutral.

Mix 85g of glycerin with 383g of ethanol properly. Remove them from the heat source and pour it into your soap mixture while simultaneously stirring vigorously using a whisk.

Pour it in gently to notice lumps of soap that form so that you can break them. To minimize the loss of ethanol, you will need to work fast. Once done, use a stick blender to break the larger pieces you couldn't break while using a whisk.

Don't be astonished if not all the soap dissolves immediately. While cooking, the lumps will then dissolve.

The fumes that will be produced from the mixture will accumulate in your room. Therefore, to protect yourself have a breathing mask on when dealing with ethanol.

Cooking Process

Place the lid back on the pot and let it cook further for approximately 45 minutes. Occasionally check the soap mixture for the temperature to be at 70° to $80^{\circ}C$. Make sure the lid is tight fitting, if not find something to secure the lid as tight as you can to avoid ethanol from escaping while cooking.

Check after 45 minutes if the soap has dissolved completely. You will notice a foamy soap layer at the top, to reduce the foam spray ethanol using your spray bottle and then use a spoon to stir. If some foam is still there, don't panic, it will dissipate in the last stage.

Sugar Syrup

To make this you will require:

Water

Sugar

Large pot

You will:

Add 113g of water to your large pot and boil it.

Turn the heat off and pour in 227g of sugar. Stir the sugar into the water to make sure it has dissolved completely.

Put back the mixture on the heat and boil it again.

When the syrup has simmered for a minute or two and all the sugar has dissolved, add the syrup to your mixture and stir as vigorously as you can.

Use a ladle to scoop the foam soap off and place it in a small bowl. Mix this and add the essential oils that you want to it. Then add a tiny amount of glycerin to the mixture and to the mold as well.

Testing the Transparency

- Use the Pyrex cup from the freezer and pour some of your clear liquid soap to it and see how transparent it is.

- At first glance, it may appear clear. But to be certain, return it to the freezer for 7 to 10 minutes then check again.

- To gauge whether you will need more solvent, the appearance of the liquid soap will be milky and totally normal.

The pot that has the mixture should be at 70°C and still cooking.

- Spray ethanol to your mixture, place the lid back on to prevent loss of ethanol when conducting your test.

- Add small doses of ethanol repeatedly and dissolved sugar as well until you achieve the transparency level you want. Depending on your sea level (SpongeBob reference), you might need to add little doses of glycerin too.

- Once transparency has been achieved, pour your soap into a jar to cool off then strain it to ensure no soap fleck or foam is in the last soap you get. The jar should be covered with a saran wrap and place the thermometer into the mixture. Let the mixture cool off to about $60^{\circ}C$, add the fragrance oils and colors.

Molding

- Now you pour the soap into your molds. If skin forms while the soap is in the molds, simply spray some ethanol to it and mix it gently to dissolve the skin immediately. Ethanol can be used in case there is any foam on the soap when you have put it in the molds.

- Place the molds in the freezer; the soap will be more transparent if it cools faster. You can remove the soap from the mold if it has hardened enough. Take it from the cool spot and place wait for a few minutes till you have to remove it from the mold.

Do not under any circumstance touch the soap with your hands, you'll leave fingerprints on the soap.

- Allow the soap to cure for two weeks and you will notice the soap becoming more transparent and harder. Polish with ethanol if skin forms on the soap then wrap it with saran to keep the humidity away.

And this is the complete process of making your transparent soap. It would look like this:

Chapter 12: Cold Process Recipes

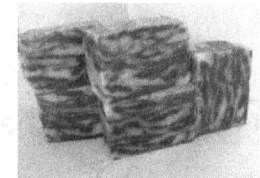

Soap with grated cocoa and carrot juice

- Cocoa oil - 35 g. (5.0%)

- Castor oil - 140 g. (20.0%)

- Coconut oil T m = 24.4 C - 70 g. (10.0%)

- Macadamia oil - 70 g. (10.0%)

- Palm kernel oil - 350 g. (50.0%)

- Vittelaria (Shea) oil - 35 g. (5.0%)

- Alkalis NaOH - 102,5 g. (superfat 8%)

- Carrot juice - 266.0 g.

- As part of the mass grated cocoa - 35 g, a bag of vanilla

- The second part - the essential oil of orange - 20 oz.

Preparation

1) Drown solid oils over the water bath (cocoa, coconut, palm kernel, shea).

2) Measure 102.5 g. of alkali.

3) Measure 266.0 g. of carrot juice (freshly squeezed)

4) Add alkali gradually into juice (not vice versa), stirring with a wooden or plastic spoon.

5) When an alkaline solution and oil reach about 40 degrees, pour alkaline solution in the oil,

 still continuing to stir.

6) After the mixture becomes turbid, blend it with mixer until the light trace appears.

7) Divide the mass into two parts:

add chocolate liquor melted over the water bath - 35g to the 1st part, a bag of vanilla

add orange essential oil - 20 g to the 2nd part.

8) Fill the two masses in the molds alternately with spoon. Wrap it in a towel for the soap passes the gel phase.

9) After 3 days (soap of juice freezes longer) we get it out from the molds and cut, set to ripen in a ventilated area for 4-6 weeks. Before using check ph soap.

Soap has a light aroma of chocolate and orange, very solid and has excellent foaming properties.

Castile soap

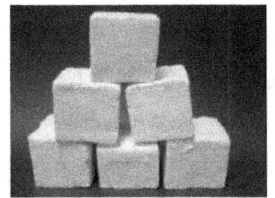

Castile soap can be non flavored - it will have the smell of bread

- 80% olive oil

- 10% of palm oil

- 10% coconut oil

You will need the following ingredients to prepare about 2 kg of soap:

- 1200 g. of olive oil

- 150 g. of palm oil

- 150 g. of coconut oil

- 450 grams of water

- Alkalis NaOH - 196,5 grams (7% superfat)

- 40-80 g. fragrance or essential oil, in accordance with your preferences

Palm oil and coconut oil is added into the recipe to make the soap hard and stable foaming. There are not many so the soap retains substantially all the properties of the true Castile.

Soap with grape juice and powdered grape seeds

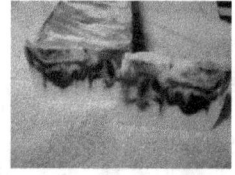

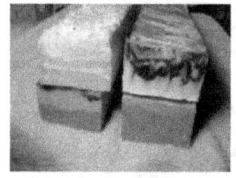

- Grape seed oil: 100 g. - 15%

- Castor oil: 40 g. - 6%

- Coconut oil T m = 24.4 C: 80 g. - 12%

- Corn oil: 100 g. - 15%

- Palm oil: 330 g.- 51%

The total weight of oils: 650 g.

- Water: 220.0 g.

- Alkali (NaOH): 85.7 g. (including 8% of superfat)

- Grape juice-fresh 30 g.

- Minced grape seeds - 2 tablespoons

- Perfume Floresans "Dark grape" - 5% - 32 g.

- In the light part - titanium dioxide.

Peculiarities of soap

- Hardness (36-50) - 39

- Cleaning (15-20) - 3

- Conditioning (45-80) - 59

- Foaminess (14-30) - 14

- Foam creaminess (16-35) - 36

- Iodine number (50) - 72

- INS (145-165) - 132

Preparation

1. Add fragrance to the oil before mixing with an alkaline solution.

2. After the "trace" appears divide the mass into 2 parts. Add juice of dark grapes, ground grape seeds into one part and add dissolved titanium dioxide (0.5 tsp.) in water (1 tablespoon) into another part.

Soap with orange peel and grated cocoa

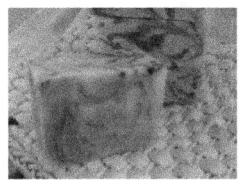

- Castor oil: 80 g. - 10%

- Coconut oil T m = 24.4 C: 80 g. - 10%

- Flaxseed oil: 80 g. - 10%

- Milk fat (cow): 160 g.- 20%

- Olive oil: 160 g. - 20%

- Chi (shea) oil: 240 g. - 30%

The total weight of oils: 800 g.

- Water: 304.0 g.

- Superfat (no need to add): 12.0%

- Alkali (NaOH): 100.3 g.

Features of soap

- Hardness (36-50) - 36

- Cleaning (15-20) - 5

- Conditioning (45-80) - 57

- Foaminess (14-30) - 19

-Foam creaminess (16-35) - 36

- Iodine number (50) - 68

- INS (145-165) - 131

Caring additives: essential oil of orange 50g, minced 2 tbsp orange zest, 1 tbsp of sea buckthorn oil, cocoa mass 30 g., cooked over the structured water.

Properties of ingredients

It provides a tonic effect. Orange oil stimulates the regeneration of dry skin, moisturizes and enhances blood circulation.

Shredded peel of citrus fruit, either orange, lemon or grapefruit is the ideal tool for peeling.

The active substances contained in the cocoa mass, help maintain skin barrier function and the optimal level of energy to synthesize collagen and elastin, activate metabolism. Tightens the skin, helps to eliminate stretch marks and smoothens wrinkles, protects against premature aging, helps maintain healthy skin, to extend its youth and beauty.

Anti-cellulite soap with laminaria seaweed

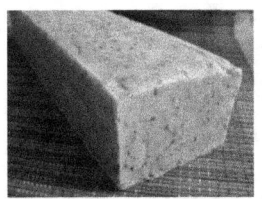

This soap moisturizes the skin, as it contains shea oil, and has a little scrub tightening effect due to algae.

- Sunflower oil - 50 g.

- Cocoa oil - 50 g.

- Castor oil - 70 g.

- Shea oil - 35 g.

- Coconut oil - 180 g.

- Olive oil - 135 g.

- Palm oil - 130 g.

The total weight of oils: 650 g.

- Alkali NaOH - 96,7 g.

- Water - 247 g.

- Superfat- shea oil - 52 g. (8%)

- Milled Laminaria seaweed about 20 g.

- Essential oils: balm and jasmine, thyme

Preparation

Algae are added just after adding superfat and essential oils. Sea salt is added into one part to enhance the improving effect.

Salt is added equally to the amount of used oils, i.e., if the mass is divided to half, then 325 g. salt must be added to the one half of the mass.

Soap with a black currant juice

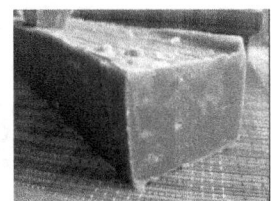

- Sunflower oil - 50 g.

- Cocoa oil - 50 g.

- Castor oil - 70 g.

- Shea oil - 35 g.

- Coconut oil - 180 g.

- Olive oil - 135 g.

- Palm oil - 130 g.

The total weight of oils: 650 g.

- Alkali NaOH - 96,7 g.

- Currant juice - 247 g.

- Superfat - grape seed oil - 52 g. (8%)

Flavors:

- Cinnamon essential oil - 20 g, orange - 20 g., neroli - 20g.

Recipe for hair soap of nettle juice

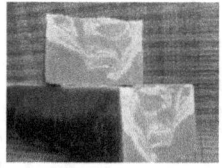

- Cocoa oil: 40 g. - 5%

- Castor oil: 120 g. - 15%

- Coconut oil T m = 24.4 C: 320 g. - 40%

- Flaxseed oil: 40 g. - 5%

- Olive oil: 40 g. - 5%

- Palm oil: 80 g. - 10%

- Sunflower oil: 80 g. - 10%

- Camelina oil: 40 g. - 5%

- Vittelaria (shea) oil: 40 g. - 5%

The total weight of oils: 800 g.

- Nettle juice - 304.0 g.

- Alkali (NaOH) - 123.0 g. considering superfat - 5.0%

Flavours:

- Neroli oil – 20 ml

- Bergamot oil – 6ml

- Lemon oil – 3 ml

- Mandarin oil – 3 ml

- Lactic acid 2% - 16 g.

Peculiarities of soap

- Hardness (36-50) - 45

- Cleansing (15-20) - 8

- Conditioning (45-80) - 50

- Foaminess (14-30) - 40

- Foam creaminess (16-35) - 31

- Iodine number (up to 50) - 61

- INS (145-165) - 160

Preparation

Nettle leaves must be carefully washed and dried to make juice. Scroll nettles through the grinder, squeeze the juice through cheesecloth. To scroll the leaves through a meat grinder easily, you should first boil them.

It's better to gather nettles in May-June, then nettle is juicier and it is easy to squeeze out its juice.

Add alkali gradually into the frozen nettle juice, stirring constantly. Drown oils over the water bath. When the oil and the alkaline solution are of the same temperature, pour the solution into the oil, wait until "trace" appears then add esters and lactic acid.

Add glycerol dissolved in titanium to the 1/3 of the mass. Pour a dark piece of soap into the mold and pour the light soap from above, mixing the top layer with the bottom a little. Align the top with a spatula. Wrap the soap, and leave it until the gel stage.

Soap is firm, foams well, rinses hair well. Many people do not like the existence of palm oil in the recipe, but I recommend adding a little to the soap for thin hair type, soap with it thickens and adds volume to hair.

Soap with floral swirls

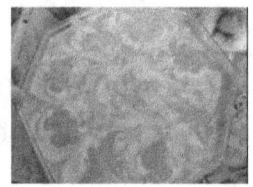

- Cocoa oil - 10%

- Palm oil - 30%

- Coconut oil – 10%

- Shea oil - 10%

- Olive oil - 40%

- Alkali, water on conversion

- Essential oil of lemon, lavender, geranium

Additional ingredients:

- yellow part - sea buckthorn oil, honey

- green part - green clay, ground dry nettle

Preparation

Heat the oil over the bath. Pour alkali into ice water, stirring gently. When the oil and the alkaline solution are of about 40C degrees (the optimal temperature, if assumed to swirl, then the mass slowly turns into the "trace"). Mix it with blender until the light "trace" appears. Add ether. We divide the mass into 3 portions of 300 grams (approximately). Part 1 - 100 grams (add lilac cosmetic pigment). 1 part of 300 grams - leave without anything, Part 1 - add sea buckthorn oil, honey, green part - green clay, ground nettles.

Pour the mass with a tablespoon into the marked areas (we have assumed 9 flowers) alternating colors - green, on top in the middle of each flower one tablespoon of yellow then in each - a spoonful of white, and finally, in the middle of a spoonful of lilac mass.

Then with a sushi stick make decor either in the middle of the flower, or from the middle to the edges. Sprinkle the top with alcohol to avoid soda ash (white patches on the soap).

Shaving Soap

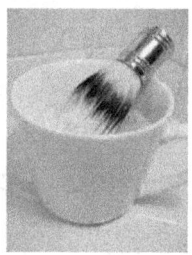

Shaving soap preparation process is almost indistinguishable from ordinary cold pulping soap method, except for the use of bentonite clay and a high percentage of castor oil in the compound, which gives abundant dense foaming.

Clay makes soap slide, has a mild effect, and is also able to deduce fat from the deep layers of skin, toxins, anti-inflammatory, absorbing and regenerating effect, which is a characteristic of mud therapy.

I prefer bentonite clay, although you can use kaolin or other clay. For 900 g. Of oils, take 2 tbsp. of clay.

Recipe:

40% Olive oil - stable foam, conditioning, softness

30% Coconut oil – rich in foam, soap hardness

22% Palm Oil - stability, hardness (can be substituted by pork fat)

8% castor oil - creamy foam

For 926 g

360 gr of olive oil

270 gr of coconut oil

Palm oil - 198 gr

72 g of castor oil

The total weight of oils: 900 g.

Alkali (NaOH) - 128,8 (5% of superfat)

Water - 270 g. (30%)

2 tablespoons of bentonitic clay

30-40 g. of essential oil

Preparation:

Cooking soap by cold method, clay and esters should be added. It's convenient to pour this soap directly into a soap dish, and you can make a common soap in any mold.

Tea with milk

Scented mint oil, orange, anise and cloves. The smell is very nice, versatile, invigorating. Soap made by cold pulping method with milk instead of water.

Recipe:

- Corn oil - 100 g (10%)

- Olive oil 500 g (50%)

- Palm oil 400 g (40%)

- Essential oils (peppermint, clove, orange, anise) - 40 ml.

- Alkali 138 g.

- Frozen milk 380 g.

- Superfat - 8% olive oil (80 g)

- Green tea powder - 4 tbsp.

Peculiarities of a milk soap.

For first milk is necessary to freeze, gradually adding alkali to milk, then stir gently.

Since the milk was frozen, so the solution is heated only to 35 degrees, you need to consider this when preparing oil. Melt the oil in advance, so they have time to cool down to 35 degrees.

Then, as usual, pour the alkaline solution in oil, stirring until the "trace" appears.

Then add superfat, essential oils. Add tea powder to one part of the soap, mix well, pour several various layers and decorate as you wish.

You can make swirls here, as you have made thin streaks by "hanger". Gel should not get to the bottom to make the lowest part of the soap as light as possible.

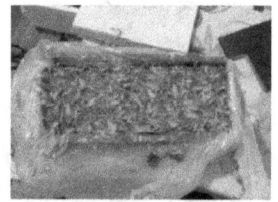

Chocolate soap

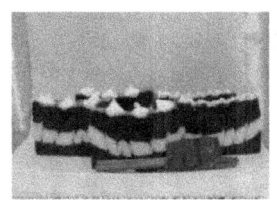

- Cocoa oil - 70 g. (10%)

- Castor oil - 140 g. (20%)

- Coconut oil - 105 g. (15%)

- Corn oil – 105 g. (15%)

- Olive oil - 70 g. (10%)

- Palm oil - 210 g. (30%)

- Alkali NaOH - 100 g.

- Structured water - 266 g. (38%)

Additives to "trace":

- Chocolate - 50 g.

- Superfat -70 g. - Olive oil (10%)

- Sodium lactate, 8.4 g (2%)

Preparation:

1) Melt solid oil over the hot water bath. Then pour liquid oils.

2) Measure 100 grams of alkali.

3) Measure 266.0 grams of very cold water

4) Carefully pour alkali into the water (not vice versa), stirring with a wooden or plastic spoon.

5) When an alkaline solution and oil are of the same temperature at the range of 40 to 60 degrees, pour alkaline solution stirring into the oil. I mixed it at 40 degrees.

6) After the mixture got turbid beat it with a mixer or blender until the "trace" appears

7) Then, add superfat, sodium lactate.

8) Pour 2/3 of mass into a container of grated and melted chocolate.

Mix well until you get a single colored mass.

You can add titanium dioxide into the rest 1/3 of the mass (a little less than 1/2 tsp.) pre-mix it with a small amount of oil to avoid grains in the soap beforehand.

9) Fill in the mold with layers. Make swirls by the method of "hanger".

To do this, take a thicker wire, shape it in the form of the so-called hanger, drive it up - down, take the mass along the entire length of the mold, for the swirls would be visible through the cuttings.

Bend the wire so as it reaches narrow side walls to maximum. Move wire up and down each time by shifting two or less, or more cm. parallel to the side wall. So the wire will take all the positions at the bottom of the mold marked with red lines.

You can decorate the top with the help of a pastry bag.

Wrap in a towel for the soap passes the gel phase or place in the turned off preheated oven.

10) One day later - remove the three pieces from the molds and cut, leave to ripen in a ventilated area for 4-6 weeks.

Beer Soap

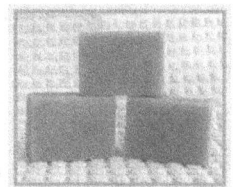

- Avocado oil - 180 g.

- Coconut oil - 270 g.

- Castor oil - 45 g.

- Olive oil - 270 g.

- Shea oil - 135 g.

The total weight of oils: 900 g.

- Beer - 324 g.

- NaOh - 126.3 g. (Superfat 5%)

Essential oil before placing them in the mold:

- Orange oil - 15 ml.

- Lemongrass oil - 15 ml.

- Palmarosa oil - 5 ml.

- Littsea oil (smell: refreshing, warm, sweet-sour, lemon-orange) - 2.5 ml.

This is a wonderful recipe for soap, beer is used instead of water, due to which the soap has rich foam.

A few days before making the soap heat up the beer without boiling it, then cool it.

Pour it in a glass bowl, cover with a lid, but not tight, for the beer ran out of steam. Before making it, put it in the fridge for the night, so it cools, and then cook as in a usual cold way.

Honey soap

You can make a very beautiful face soap like honeycombs with an oilcloth with air bubbles, which is often used to wrap gadgets to protect from damage. You can find such oilcloth in a hardware store.

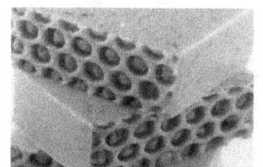

- Castor oil - 75 g.

- Coconut oil - 75 g.

- Palm oil - 315 g.

The total weight of oils: 465 g.

- Alkali NaOH - 68,1 g.

- Decoction of calendula - 176.7 g. (38%)

- Superfat - olive oil 35 g. (7%)

- 1 tablespoon honey

- 1 tablespoon dried calendula petals.

- 20 g. essential oils (jasmine and myrrh).

Preparation:

1. Drown 465.0 g. of oil over a hot bath,

2. Measure 68.1 g. of alkali.

3. Measure 176.7 g. of very cold decoction.

4. Gently pour alkali into the water (not vice versa), stirring with a wooden or plastic spoon.

5. When the alkaline solution and the oil will be the same temperature at the range of 40 to 60 degrees, pour alkaline solution in the oil stirring gently.

6. After the mixture gets turbid, mix it with a mixer or blender until the "trace" appears, like on photo.

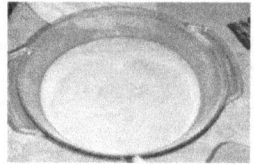

7. Then 35.0 g. of olive oil (superfat) should be added to the honey, calendula petals, dyes, essential oils.

8. At the bottom of the mold put a pellicle with bubbles. Pour mass into the mold. Wrap it in a towel for the soap passes the gel phase.

9. The next day take it out of the mold and cut, leave to ripen in a ventilated area for 4-6 weeks.

Soap turned dark thanks to honey, calendula petals are almost invisible on this background, the soap foams perfectly (large, airy foams), well softens the skin, does not dry the skin, and of course has a nice spicy flavor.

Oatmeal soap

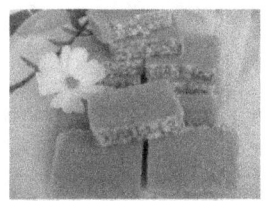

- Palm oil -300 g.

- Coconut oil - 200 g.

- Olive oil - 200 g.

- Cocoa oil -100 g.

- Palm kernel oil - 100g

- Castor Oil - 50 oz.

- Sesame oil - 50 g.

The total weight of oils: 1000 g.

- Alkali NaOH - 143,45 g.

- Oatmeal (instead of water) – 380 g.

After the gel stage add:

- Superfat - 50 g. (5%)

- Crushed oatmeal - 100 g.

- Silkworm cocoons -10 pieces.

Silk proteins help moisturize the skin and make the foam softer and velvety.

Oatmeal provides many good effects to the skin, including cleansing effect, deeply nourishes and makes the skin soft and velvety. Oats is a great beautician and if you use oatmeal soap every morning, you will forget about the skin problems. Oat flakes, milled into flour, peel off, soothen and deeply penetrate into the skin layers, clean the epidermis well.

Conclusion

Thank you again for downloading this book!

I hope this book was able to help you learn how to make soaps and will help you enjoy this craft. I also hope it will encourage those who wish to turn soap making into a business to take action and make it happen. The world is waiting to experience your creativity.

There are a lot of special oils, essential oils and other add-in ingredients which you can add to your soaps. There are also a hundred ways you can design your soaps. I encourage you to start experimenting with soap making and see where this exciting craft will take you.

www.ingramcontent.com/pod-product-compliance
Lightning Source LLC
Chambersburg PA
CBHW071826080526
44589CB00012B/924